GP REFERRAL SCHEMES

DEBBIE LAWRENCE AND LOUISE BARNETT
WORKING WITH GP-REFERRED CLIENTS

A & C BLACK · LONDON

Thanks to Fitness Professionals Ltd (www.fitpro.com) for supporting the Fitness Professionals series.

Published in 2006 by A & C Black Publishers Ltd
38 Soho Square, London W1D 3HB
www.acblack.com

ISBN-10: 0 7136 7707 4
ISBN-13: 978 0 7136 7707 2

A CIP record for this book is available from the British Library.

Acknowledgements
Cover photograph © Corbis
Illustrations by Jean Ashley

Printed and bound in Great Britain by Biddles Ltd, King's Lynn.

CONTENTS

ACKNOWLEDGEMENTS

This has been the most challenging of all the books I have researched and written. It has taught me a great deal.

The first person I would like to acknowledge is my co-author Louise Barnett who has a wealth of experience working in the fitness industry with specialist populations. I am thankful for her expertise and attention to detail, and her thorough and dedicated approach to researching the specific areas she has written and presented in this book. Her efforts have contributed considerably to the development and progress of the book.

Thanks, for proofreading and providing feed-back, to Sheena Land, Dr Bill Pomeroy from The Oaks Surgery (Kent), Keith Smith, Patrick Ogbonna (Patch) and Tessa Hicks.

As usual, thanks also to all my counselling and personal training clients.

May you all lead a happy and healthy life.

Debbie Lawrence
July 2006

I would like to thank Debbie Lawrence for giving me the opportunity to be involved in this exciting project, and for her guidance along the way.

Many thanks to friends, colleagues and clients for their ongoing support, encouragement and enthusiasm for physical activity. A very special thanks to Tony Johnston, Sheila Taylor, Keith Smith, Ruth Shaw, Amy Russell and Eric Wilmot for efforts beyond the call of duty.

Louise Barnett
July 2006

INTRODUCTION

The aim of this book is to provide an introductory practical resource for fitness instructors and personal trainers working with clients referred to exercise by their GP or other health professional. It raises awareness of some of the current guidelines and considerations that should inform exercise professionals working with clients with specific medical conditions.

It does *not* replace the need for specialist training for those who work with the specific groups and special populations addressed in this book, *nor* does it replace the need to consult with a medical expert regarding the use of exercise as part of a self-management/treatment plan.

It is *not* the ultimate textbook or education reference for specific medical conditions. A compendium of other resources has been researched and referenced to inform the contents. The book aims to introduce some medical conditions and discuss these at a level deemed by the writers to be a sufficient starting point for an exercise professional to develop his or her knowledge and experience.

The strength of the book is that it makes recommendations and offers suggestions based on current research and information on how to adapt exercise to enable participation by special groups. The intention is to provide basic guidance, but in all instances the specific needs and requirements of the individual, together with any other relevant factors, should be considered and accounted for before making any exercise recommendation. In many instances, referred clients present with multiple rather than isolated conditions.

With this in mind, any exercise recommendation *must* be tailored for the individual with reference to all of his or her specific conditions and existing abilities and needs. Consultation with the client's GP regarding the frequency, intensity, time and type of exercise to be administered is also an essential factor in planning an individual schedule.

LIST OF ABBREVIATIONS

1RM	1 repetition maximum
6MWT	6-minute walk test
ABPM	Ambulatory blood pressure
ADL	Activity of daily living
AED	Automated external defibrillator
BDZ	Benzodiazepine
BMI	Body mass index
BP	Blood pressure
bpm	Beats per minute
CABG	Coronary artery bypass graft
CBA	Cerebrovascular accident
CHD	Coronary heart disease
CNS	Central nervous system
COPD	Chronic obstructive pulmonary disease
CPSP	Central post-stroke pain
CVD	Cardiovascular disease
DBP	Diastolic blood pressure
DMARD	Disease-modifying anti-rheumatic drug
ECG	Electrocardiogram
ECT	Electroconvulsive therapy
EELV	End-expiratory lung volume
EIA	Exercise-induced asthma
FEV	Forced expiratory volume
FITT	Frequency, intensity, time and type
FVC	Forced vital capacity
GAD	General anxiety disorder
GTN	Glyceryl trinitate

HbA1c	Haemoglobin A1c
HDL	High-density lipoproteins
HR	Heart rate
HRT	Hormone replacement therapy
HRR	Heart rate reserve
HRmax	Maximal heart rate
IDP	Idiopathic Parkinson's disease
IFG	Impaired fasting glycaemia
IGT	Impaired glucose tolerance
ISWT	Incremental shuttle walk test
IVIg	Intravenous immunoglobin
LDL	Low-density lipoproteins
LTOT	Long-term oxygen therapy
MET	Metabolic equivalent
MHR	Maximum heart rate
MI	Myochardial infarction
mmol/l	Millimoles per litre
MOAI	Monoamine oxidase inhibitor
MRI	Magnetic resonance imaging
MS	Multiple sclerosis
NIDDM	Non-insulin-dependent diabetes mellitus
NQAF	National Quality Assurance Framework
NRT	Nicotine replacement therapy
OGTT	Oral glucose tolerance test
PaO$_2$	Partial pressure of oxygen (in arterial blood)

PCI	Percutaneous coronary intervention
PD	Parkinson's disease
PEF	Peak expiratory flow
PNF	Proprioreceptive neuromuscular facilitation
PTSD	Post-traumatic stress disorder
rep	Repetition
REPs	Register of Exercise Professionals
ROM	Range of motion/movement
RPE	Rating of perceived exertion
rpm	Revolutions per minute
SAH	Subarachnoid haemorrhage
SD	Standard deviation
SPB	Systolic blood pressure
spm	Strokes per minute
SSRI	Specific stress-related disorder
THR	Training heart rate
TIA	Transient ischaemic attack
TLCO	Transfer factor for carbon dioxide
TPR	Total peripheral resistance
VO$_2$Max	Maximum volume of oxygen
VO$_2$R	Volume of oxygen reserve

PHYSICAL ACTIVITY, EXERCISE AND HEALTH

PART **ONE**

The Chief Medical Officer (DOH 2005*a*) reveals that levels of physical activity in the British population have declined in recent decades to a level that impacts health and well-being.

To overgeneralise and perhaps overexaggerate the issues, as a nation we are *suffering* in numerous ways and at many levels:

- **Physically** Compared to previous generations, we walk less, cycle less, drive more, drive or use public transport unnecessarily (short journeys and school runs), spend more time watching television and DVDS, spend more time playing with computer games and home technology, and our lifestyles (work, home and leisure) are more sedentary.
- **Nutritionally** We eat more fast, processed and convenience food, eat insufficient fruit and vegetables, eat too many foods high in sugar and fat, consume too much coffee and tea, drink too little water.
- **Socially** We drink alcohol more regularly, smoke more, and increasingly use illegal drugs for recreational purposes. There are more fast-food restaurants. There are less safe places to be active (parks and fields). Levels of obesity are increasing, especially among children and young people.
- **Mentally and emotionally** Lifestyles are fast-paced. Self-esteem is lower. Stress, depression, anxiety and other mental health conditions are more prevalent.
- **Medically** The levels of chronic diseases such as diabetes, high blood pressure, high cholesterol, stroke, coronary heart disease, depression and obesity are increasing, and the demands on the NHS are stretched.
- **Spiritually** There are wars and riots, prejudice, intolerance to diversity and difference, power struggles in relationships and a general lack of community.

The whole picture creates a sorry story indeed, especially for a nation of people that can be considered one of the most privileged in the world!

This section of the book introduces and explains the value of physical activity as a method for improving health and refers to publications defining specific government strategies for further reading. It also discusses the concept of exercise and the components of physical fitness, and provides generalised ideas on how to adapt exercise intensity for persons of a lower fitness level. (Condition-specific considerations are discussed in Part Three.) It also introduces the components of total fitness as a model of health and discusses the impact of other lifestyle factors on health.

PHYSICAL ACTIVITY

Physical activity is the umbrella term used for any human movement that results in an increase in energy expenditure above resting level. This includes activities of everyday living such as:

- getting dressed
- active hobbies and leisure pursuits
- housework
- gardening
- walking or cycling instead of other forms of transport
- climbing stairs instead of using escalators and lifts
- manual labour tasks
- exercising
- sporting activities.

Current levels of physical activity

There are numerous opportunities for being more physically active at home and at work, during leisure time and in the way in which we travel. However, the reality is that the majority of people are inactive and do comparatively little physical activity (DoH 2004a), with people in lower socio-economic groups generally showing lower activity levels than people from other groups. The Joint Health Surveys Unit, in its reports Health Survey for England (2003) and the Health of Minority Ethnic Groups (1999) estimates that:

- 6 out of 10 men are not active enough to benefit their health;
- 7 out of 10 women are not active enough to benefit their health;

- people become less active as they get older;
- South Asian and Chinese women and men are less likely to participate in physical activities of all kinds;
- Bangladeshi men and women are the least physically active.

In developed countries there has been a decline in the levels of physical activity. This is due to a number of factors including:

- increased use of cars for short journeys such as driving to a local train station and taking children to school;
- perception of the environment as being unsafe for children to play outside the home (parks and fields);
- increase in sedentary leisure and play activities including television and computer games;
- decreased participation in sport;
- reduced opportunities for physical activity and sporting activities within the school curriculum.

Most people are affected in some way by these trends and it is often seen as increasingly difficult for people to maintain optimal levels of physical activity.

Benefits of physical activity

There is substantial evidence to support the role of physical activity in promoting and managing health. The Chief Medical Officer's report 'At Least Five a Week' reinforces the link between lack of physical activity and ill health and establishes the importance of physical activity as a major causal factor for guarding against chronic disease (Department of Health 2004).

The report claims that physically active adults have:

- 20–30 per cent reduced risk of premature death;
- up to 50 per cent reduced chance of developing diseases such as coronary heart disease (CHD), stroke, diabetes and certain cancers;
- improved functional capacity;
- reduced risk of back pain;
- increased independence (older people);
- increased bone density and reduced risk of osteoporosis;
- improved psychological well-being;
- reduced risk of stress and anxiety;
- reduced risk of clinical depression;
- reduced risk of falls (older adults);
- improved weight loss and weight management.

Physical activity features in many recent government policies and initiatives as a medium for improving health. These include:

- The National Quality assurance framework (DoH 2001*a*)
- *Saving Lives: Our Healthier Nation* (DoH 1999*a*)
- NHS Plan (DoH 2000*b*)
- *National Service Frameworks* (NSFs) which include: *Mental Health* (DoH 1999*b*), *CHD* (DoH 2000*a*), *Cancer* (DoH 2000*c*), *Older People* (DoH 2001*d*), *Diabetes* (DoH 2001*c*), *Children* (DoH 2004*c*)
- Chief Medical Officer (CMO) (DoH 2003*a*) annual report, *On the State of Public Health*
- Healthy schools (www.wiredforhealth.gov.uk)
- *Tackling Health Inequalities: A Programme for Action* (DoH 2003*b*)
- *Choosing Health* (DoH 2004*b*)
- *At Least Five a Week* (DoH 2004*a*).

Readers are referred to the British Heart Foundation and Sport England (2005*e*) summary brief on *Physical Activity and Health* and other Department of Health strategies, as referenced for further information.

Recommended levels of physical activity for adults

The current recommendations for physical activity to maintain general health were set out in the *Strategy Statement on Physical Activity* by the Department of Health (1996). These targets are outlined in table 1.1.

Barriers to physical activity

Barriers or blocks to being more active can be classified as either intrinsic or extrinsic. Intrinsic barriers relate to how the individual feels about physical activity. This will be influenced by their past experiences (in school, with family etc.) and their beliefs concerning physical activity (instilled by education, family, socialisation) which can influence both interest in physical activity and confidence to take part. Extrinsic barriers relate to broader issues such as access to and availability of appropriate and affordable physical activity (i.e. in leisure centres, community centres, activity groups), the environment (safety of roads, parks, concerns for personal security, etc.), opportunities for physical activity (at work, school, home) and the attitude and skills of other people (exercise professionals, family, teachers, health professionals, etc.).

The Department of Health (2004*b*), 'Choosing Health', and the Health Development Agency (2005*a*) report on 'The Effectiveness of Public Health Interventions for Increasing Physical Activity amongst Adults' both cite other social factors that influence participation in sport and

Table 1.1	Targets for physical activity
Frequency	Work towards building activity into daily routine on 5 days of the week (minimum)
Intensity	Work at a moderate level where you feel mildly breathless, warm but comfortable
Time	Work towards performing the chosen activities for a total of 30 minutes. This can be broken down and accumulated, for example: 3 × 10-minute slots of activity each day 2 × 15-minute slots of activity each day
Type	Any activity that fits well into your daily lifestyle! For example: Walking to the station Walking the kids to school Vigorous housework Cleaning the car Walking up and down stairs more frequently Dancing to a piece of music at home Active hobbies Structured exercise and sporting activities A combination of activity, exercise and sport

This recommendation can be tailored specifically to the lifestyle, preference and needs of the individual and is particularly relevant for the people who find it easier and more acceptable to increase physical activity by incorporating it into their everyday life. |

exercise. These include lower levels of physical activity being reported among the following categories of the population:

• some minority ethnic groups
• people in low-income households
• lower social classes
• people with lower levels of educational attainment
• people performing non-professional and non-managerial status work
• older people.

The latter of these reports specifically addresses the need for future research to examine these social determinants further.

People of any age, ethnicity and gender etc. will experience certain barriers to activity and exercise, which may include a lack of:

• money (cost)
• interest
• confidence
• time
• motivation

or a prioritisation of other responsibilities (children, family, work, etc.).

Older people may face additional barriers. These may include:

- fear of overdoing it, injuring themselves or aggravating a medical condition;
- embarrassment and feeling they don't fit in or wouldn't be able to keep up;
- safety concerns, such as a fear of falling in some environments (e.g. swimming pools);
- lack of culturally appropriate facilities.

(BHF 2003*a*)

Risks associated with health-related physical activity

The benefits of physical activity are substantial and far outweigh the risks associated with participation. Many of the risks associated with physical activity can be avoided.

The following groups are usually at the greatest risk from injury. People who:

- do too much exercise;
- take part in vigorous activity or competitive sport;
- do too much too soon;
- have an existing condition or disease that may require an adapted programme.

People who do too much exercise are rare; however, there are individuals who become obsessive about exercise. They will experience withdrawal symptoms if they have an injury or social engagement that prevents them from exercising. This obsessive behaviour is not caused by exercise, but is more likely to be connected to an underlying psychological disorder and/or maybe an addictive tendency within the personality. For example, people

with eating disorders such as anorexia nervosa may use exercise as a way to control weight.

Promoting physical activity

Evidence shows that the people who are most likely to benefit from an increase in physical activity are the least active. All the government initiatives have been set out to promote physical activity at a national and local level.

When working with individuals to promote physical activity, it is important that any increase in activity levels starts at a low and steady level and progresses very gradually in relation to frequency, intensity and time. There are various factors to consider to promote participation in physical activity. Some of these are listed in table 1.2.

How personal trainers and exercise professionals can help

Personal trainers and exercise professionals can contribute to improving activity levels by promoting activity at every opportunity. They can help to spread the activity message by:

- writing for local papers;
- working with local GP surgeries;
- speaking on local radio;
- working with local hospitals;
- taking exercise back into the community (e.g. in church halls and community centres);
- organising sessions in the workplace;
- working with local primary care trusts and other local health groups.

They can also make appropriate recommendations as to the frequency, time and type of activity for individuals to make a start towards building their activity levels and promoting healthier living.

Table 1.2	**Intrinsic and extrinsic factors to enable participation**
Intrinsic	*Extrinsic*
• Individual factors (age, gender etc.) • Previous injuries • Musculo-skeletal conditions/diseases such as arthritis • Existing disease such as CHD • Medication	• Environment, including availability of appropriate exercise spaces (safe parks etc.). The type of surface, temperature, and traffic if exercising outside. • Clothing and footwear (cycle helmet if cycling, warm clothing to exercise outside) • Level of supervision (personal training, group exercise or exercise alone) • Type of activity • Volume of activity (frequency, intensity and duration) • Session structure. The inclusion of a prolonged warm-up and cool-down is important for special populations such as older people and people with CHD

EXERCISE AND PHYSICAL FITNESS

2

Exercise

Exercise can be described as any activity that is planned, structured and performed regularly with a specific goal or purpose in mind, for example: to improve fitness and/or health. Exercise may involve going to the gym, going for a run or a swim or attending a group exercise session.

The amount of exercise people do can be described in terms of frequency, intensity, time and type or mode. The combination of frequency, intensity and time over a fixed period is referred to as the volume of exercise.

Physical fitness

Physical fitness is achieved by performing specific types of exercise in a structured format, at a recommended frequency, intensity and duration/time. There are five components of physical fitness:

- cardiovascular fitness
- flexibility
- muscular fitness (muscular strength and endurance)
- motor fitness.

Cardiovascular fitness

Cardiovascular fitness is the ability of the heart, lungs and circulatory system to transport and utilise oxygen and remove waste products efficiently. It is sometimes referred to as cardio-respiratory fitness, stamina, or aerobic fitness.

Benefits of cardiovascular training

To maintain our quality of life and ability to take part in recreational activities it is essential that we have an efficient cardiovascular system. Low cardiovascular fitness is associated with an increased risk of chronic diseases such as diabetes, high blood pressure, high cholesterol and coronary heart disease, all of which ultimately cause premature death. Increased physical activity, exercise and improved cardiovascular fitness can assist with the prevention of these diseases, promote better quality of life and reduce some of the unnecessary burden on the National Health Service that these conditions create.

Regular cardiovascular exercise enables the heart to become stronger, which allows it to pump a greater volume of blood in each contraction (stroke volume). The capillary network in the muscles and around the lungs will increase, which allows the transportation of more oxygen to the body cells and the swifter removal of waste products. The size and number of mitochondria, the cells in which aerobic energy is produced, will increase, enabling increased utilisation of oxygen. Cardiovascular training has a positive effect on overall health and specific benefits include:

- achievement and maintenance of weight loss;
- reduced risk of high blood pressure, heart disease and stroke;
- improvement in cholesterol levels;
- preventing or delaying the development of Type 2 diabetes;

- management of Type 1 and Type 2 diabetes;
- reduced risks of certain cancers.

Recommended training guidelines for developing and maintaining cardiovascular fitness are listed in table 2.1.

Adapting cardiovascular training for referred populations

The frequency, intensity, time and type of cardiovascular programme recommended should take into account a range of factors including:

- fitness level of the individual;

Table 2.1	Recommended training guidelines for cardiovascular fitness
Frequency How often should we perform these activities?	3 to 5 times a week. 3 times a week is sufficient for persons exercising at higher intensities. More than 3 times a week is recommended for people exercising at low levels of intensity.
	People with very low functional capacity may benefit from one or two short sessions per day.
	Rest days should be alternated with vigorous training days. Vary the activities and alter the impact to avoid injury to the muscles and joints.
Intensity How hard should we be working?	55/65% to 90% HRmax (heart rate max) 40/50% to 85% HRR (heart rate reserve)
	A range of 70–85% HRmax or 60–80% HR reserve is sufficient for most individuals to improve cardiovascular fitness when combined with appropriate frequency and duration.
	Lower levels of intensity are appropriate for the less active individuals; however, duration may need to be increased.
Time/Duration How long should we sustain these activities for?	For training purposes, 20–60 min of continuous or intermittent activity, e.g. accumulating 10-min bouts throughout the day.
	Minimum duration to improve cardiovascular fitness in apparently healthy adults is 20–30 min. All durations exclude necessary time for warm-up and cool-down.
	Less fit groups will need to progress gradually to increased durations.
Type/Mode/Specificity What type of activities are most effective?	Rhythmical, continuous activities that use large muscle groups e.g. walking, swimming, running, cycling, dancing, rowing, stepping.

Adapted from ACSM (2005)

- the condition(s) with which they have been referred;
- the effects of any medication on the exercise response;
- other lifestyle factors (smoking etc.);
- goal, e.g. weight loss;
- client preference.

Previously inactive people will generally have to work at a lower intensity and in order to achieve their goals they may have to increase the frequency and duration of the activity. They may also have lower levels of body awareness and muscular fitness, and their exercise technique may demand more careful attention (observation, correction, teaching) to enable safe participation. The mode of activity will need careful consideration, taking account of physical impairments or limitations such as postural instability or hemiplegia (muscle weakness on one side of the body). For example a recumbent bike or an upper extremity ergometer may be more appropriate than treadmill walking for an individual with postural instability. A client with hemiplegia may benefit from a combined upper and lower body ergometer, using the unaffected leg and arm to assist with the movement (ACSM 2005*b*).

There are specific variants that can be altered to change and adapt the intensity of specific cardiovascular exercise types/modes. These are:

- rate
- resistance
- range of motion
- repetitions
- rest.

Rate/Speed

Varying the speed at which cycling, rowing, stepping, walking and running are performed will vary the intensity of the exercise. Working at a slower pace will generally be easier than working at a faster pace. However, it is essential that the exercises remain rhythmical in nature (not too slow or too quick) in order for them to be comfortable and sustainable for an appropriate duration. As a general guideline start slower and progressively build the pace to a comfortable, sustainable level. Table 2.2 lists how speed/rate can be varied on different cardiovascular machines.

Resistance/Weight

An individual's body-weight will automatically add resistance to exercise. It will require more effort from the muscles to lift and move a heavier body-weight than a lighter one against the force of gravity. This should be considered

Table 2.2	Adapting speed using cardiovascular machines
Cardiovascular machines	*Variant: Rate/speed measure*
Rowing machine	Strokes per minute (spm)
Cycling machine	Revolutions per minute (rpm)
Treadmill	Miles per hour (mph) or kilometres per hour (kph)
Step machine	Number of steps or floors climbed
Cross trainer	Number of stride revolutions

when working with people who are overweight or obese or with persons with joint or bone conditions (osteoporosis/osteoarthritis) as even low-impact weight-bearing exercises will already be placing additional stress on their joints. In these instances, prescribed activities should ideally be of a lower impact, such as walking and, for some groups, non-weight-bearing, such as swimming or cycling. Adding propulsion or impact such as jogging on a trampette or running on a treadmill is a way of increasing intensity, but may not be appropriate for all individuals due to increased stress on the lower extremities.

Swimming and water-based exercise programmes offer greater support to the body and are comparatively less stressful on the joints. Water-based programmes demand the body to move against and through the resistance of water and require the muscles of the upper body to have a much greater involvement to create that movement. Increasing the surface area of the body or moving limbs or using buoyancy equipment (a tube/woggle, water bells, water mitts etc.) will all increase the resistance created and increase the intensity of exercises performed in water. As a general guideline, start the programme without using equipment and progress by building in the use of equipment that increases the surface area/resistance being moved.

Most gym-based cardiovascular machines (rower, cross trainer, cycle, stepper, etc.) offer a variable workload. The intensity or workload can be altered by changing the level of resistance, which can vary (usually between levels of 1 (easiest) to 20 (hardest)) depending on specific machines and manufacturers. Lower levels of resistance are generally easier and higher levels are generally harder; however, it is essential to refer to specific manufacturers' guidelines to check the level of resistance. A general guideline is to start at a lower level of resistance and progressively increase to a comfortable working level.

Repetitions/Rest

Different methods of training (continuous and interval) can be used to improve cardiovascular fitness. Continuous activity aims to maintain a specific intensity throughout a specified duration. This may not be appropriate for deconditioned individuals starting cardiovascular training, or those with specific conditions such as chronic obstructive pulmonary disease (COPD). These individuals will benefit from an interval training approach with prescribed work and rest times. For example: walking at a faster pace for an established period of time (work ratio) and then lowering the intensity for an established period time (rest ratio) to allow the person to recover. As a general guideline, starting with shorter work times, a lower number of work intervals and longer (and more frequent) rest time intervals is appropriate. Progressively increasing the duration of the work ratios and the number (frequency) of work intervals, and decreasing the time of rest intervals, will provide progression.

Range of motion

To increase or decrease the range of motion of cardiovascular activities, we have to increase the size of the movement by stepping higher, increasing the depth of a knee bend during a squat or increasing the length of a stride during travelling moves. Range of movement can also apply to the upper body during cardiovascular activity (e.g. lifting arms to waist height or above the shoulders whilst stepping sideways). As a general guideline: start with a smaller range of movement and gradually increase to ensure an appropriate progression of intensity and to reduce the risk of increased stress on the joints. It is also important to consider the speed of movement when increasing the range to avoid a compromise in technique and an increased risk of injury.

Empathy training for instructors

It can be useful for trainers and instructors to experience specific workouts with simulations of the restrictions imposed on some referred populations. (This is not always easy – many conditions cannot be simulated.) Some examples are: extra padding and weights can be worn to demonstrate the restrictions an overweight or obese person may experience when getting onto machines and working at specific intensities/impacts; restrictions could also be made to some ranges of movement of specific joints to help instructors understand limitations of movement.

Flexibility

Flexibility is the ability of our joints and muscles to move through their full potential range of movement. It is sometimes referred to as suppleness or mobility.

Benefits of flexibility

Being able to move the joints and muscles through their full potential range of motion is essential for easing the performance of all our everyday tasks. Shoulder joint flexibility is needed to reach to change a light bulb, button shirts or cardigans and reach for objects on a high shelf. Hip joint flexibility is needed to lift the knees to climb stairs and take long strides when walking. Spine mobility enables us to twist and turn. Being flexible enables us to move more efficiently and contributes to the maintenance of correct posture and joint alignment. Shortened muscles around the chest and shoulders (pectorals and anterior deltoids) and weak muscles in the upper back (trapezius and rhomboids) can lead to rounding of the upper back and the postural condition of kyphosis. Shortened and/or tight hamstrings and hip flexors and weak abdominals can lead to the postural condition of lordosis. Improved posture can potentially enhance physical appearance, reduce the incidence of low back pain and assist with the management of joint mobility conditions such as osteoarthritis and rheumatoid arthritis. Being sufficiently flexible contributes to an enhanced quality of life and reduces the risk of injury, especially for older populations. The recommended training guidelines for improving and maintaining flexibility are listed in table 2.3.

To improve flexibility, static stretching should be included in the programme. Stretching should always be performed when the muscles are warm to avoid injury. Static stretching involves the muscle being slowly lengthened to the end of the range of movement, to a point of tightness, but not discomfort. This position is then held for 15–30 seconds. To improve flexibility the stretches should be repeated 2–4 times. Proprioceptive neuromuscular facilitation (PNF) is a different type of stretching technique that is not recommended for the general population; however, it may be appropriate for specific populations. It involves a 6-second contraction followed by an assisted stretch. This technique requires a partner who is trained in PNF stretching, takes more time and is associated with increased muscle soreness. Activities such as yoga and Pilates can also be used to increase flexibility and may be appropriate for some clients (ACMS 2005). For further information about stretching, refer to the *Complete Guide to Stretching* (Norris 2004).

Table 2.3	Recommended guidelines for training flexibility
Frequency How often should we perform these activities?	A minimum of 2–3 times per week Ideally 5–7 days a week The body must be warm prior to stretching to prevent muscle tearing and to enhance the range of motion
Intensity How hard should we be working?	Stretch positions should be taken to a point of mild tension, not discomfort, and held for an extended period of time
Time/Duration How long should we sustain these activities for?	2–4 repetitions can be perfomed for each stretch Hold static for 15–30 seconds
Type/Mode/Specificity What type of activities are most effective?	Static stretches are recommended for the general population

Adapted from ACSM (2005).

Adapting flexibility training for referred populations

The intensity of stretch positions will need to correspond to the:

- range of motion of the individual (variable at each joint);
- condition(s) with which the person has been referred;
- effects of any medication on the exercise response;
- other lifestyle factors.

Previously inactive people and people with specific joint and muscular problems may lack flexibility and will therefore need more supportive and comfortable positions. They may also have less body awareness and their exercise technique may demand more careful attention (observation, correction, teaching) to enable safe participation.

There are specific variants that can be altered to change and adapt the intensity of specific stretches. These are:

- range of motion
- balance
- isolation.

Range of motion

Less flexible participants will generally need to work through a smaller range of motion. Static and passive stretches in supported positions will offer them greater control for performing the stretch and achieving an appropriate range of motion.

Using gravity to assist the stretch, using towels to support levers (quadriceps and hamstring stretch), and trainer-assisted stretches (if appropriate) can be used to help the range of motion and support the stretch position. (See Fig. 2.1.)

Balance

It may also be necessary to adapt some stretch positions for less flexible people and people

Figure 2.1

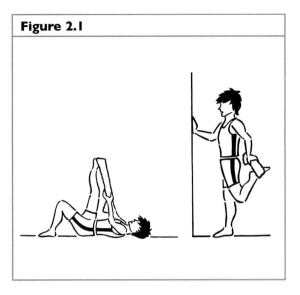

with low muscular fitness who may be unable to hold some positions.

Using a wall to provide balance, using floor-based positions (if the person has sufficient

Figure 2.2

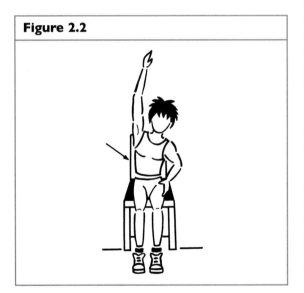

functional mobility), and using chair-based stretch positions are all appropriate ways to adapt stretch positions and assist performance. (See Fig. 2.2.)

Isolation

Isolating stretches and using easier positions are more appropriate techniques than using stretch positions where multiple muscles are stretched. It is hard to find stretches that totally isolate one muscle; however, some traditional stretch positions are much harder and demand greater flexibility of other muscles and greater work to hold the position than other stretch positions. When working with persons with low levels of flexibility, it is essential to find the most comfortable and supportive position for them.

Muscular fitness (strength and endurance)

Muscular fitness is a combination of and a balance between muscular strength and muscular endurance and represents the functional fitness needed to maintain correct posture and perform daily activities. Muscular strength is the ability of our muscles to exert a near maximal force to lift a resistance. Muscular endurance requires a less maximal force to be exerted, but for the muscle contraction to be maintained for a longer duration.

Benefits of muscular fitness training

Muscles need to be strong enough and have sufficient endurance to carry out daily tasks, which require us to lift, carry, pull or push a resistance. These may include carrying shopping, gardening, moving furniture, climbing stairs and lifting our body to/from a chair or into/out of a bath.

Strong muscles will help us to maintain the correct alignment of our skeleton. Weakened muscles may cause an uneven pull to be placed on our skeleton. Our muscles work in pairs (as one contracts and works, the opposite muscle relaxes). Therefore, any imbalance in workload (if one of the pair is contracted or worked too frequently and becomes too strong and the other is not worked sufficiently or is allowed to become weaker) will cause the joints to be pulled out of the correct alignment. This may potentially cause injury, or create postural defects such as rounded shoulders or excessive curvatures of the spine. These are illustrated in Fig. 2.3.

An imbalance of strength between the abdominal and opposing muscles of the back (the erector spinae) can cause an exaggerated curve or hollowing of the lumbar vertebrae (lordosis). An imbalance of strength between the muscles of the chest (the pectorals) and the muscles between the shoulder blades (the rhomboids and trapezii) can cause rounded shoulders and a humping of the thoracic spine (kyphosis). An imbalance in strength between the muscles on each side of the back can cause a sideways curvature of the thoracic spine (scoliosis). All muscles should therefore be kept sufficiently strong to maintain a correct posture.

Lifestyle may demand that we specifically target certain muscles more than others to compensate for imbalances caused by our work and daily activities. For the majority of persons with a sedentary lifestyle, it is well worth while strengthening the abdominal muscles, the muscles in between the shoulder blades (trapezius and rhomboids), and possibly the muscles of the back (erector spinae) and stretching the opposing muscles to these groups (pectorals, erector spinae, hip flexors and hamstrings).

Training for muscular fitness will improve the tone of our muscles and provide a firmer and

Figure 2.3 Curvatures of the spine

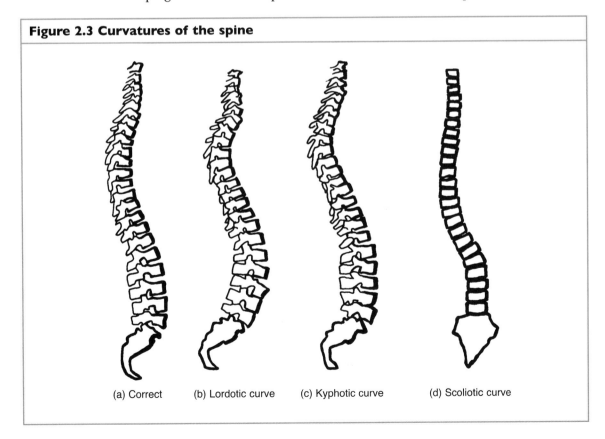

(a) Correct   (b) Lordotic curve   (c) Kyphotic curve   (d) Scoliotic curve

more shapely appearance. This can contribute to a positive self-image and can enhance psychological well-being and self-confidence.

Muscular fitness improves the strength and health of our bones and joints. The muscles have to contract and pull against the bones to create movement and lift the resistance. In response, our tendons, which attach the muscles to the bone across the joint, and our ligaments, which attach bone to bone across the joint, will become stronger. Therefore, in the long term our joints will become stronger, more stable and at less risk from injury. In addition, increased calcium can be deposited and stored by the bones. This can prevent them from becoming brittle and reduce the risk of osteoporosis. Muscular fitness training can therefore provide many long-lasting benefits that can extend the quality of our life for a number of years. The recommended training

Table 2.4	Recommended guidelines for training muscular fitness
Frequency How often should we perform these activities?	2–3 times per week (same muscle groups) for muscular fitness Alternate rest and training days (not consecutive days)
Intensity How hard should we be working?	To the point of near fatigue, while maintaining good technique For people with health conditions, finish the exercise when the lifting phase becomes difficult, while maintaining good technique
Time/duration How long should we sustain these activities for?	1 set of 3–20 reps Choose a range of reps e.g. 3–5, 10–12, 12–15 1 set of 8–12 (high intensity) will elicit strength and endurance benefits for healthy populations 1 set of 10–15 (moderate intensity) is recommended for older adults Training time will vary depending on the level of fitness, number of exercises and muscle groups and fitness goals
Type/mode/specificity What type of activities are most effective?	8–10 exercises targeting the main muscle groups Choose activities that are comfortable throughout the range of movement Free weights Resistance machines Body-weight exercises Body bars Exercise bands

Adapted from ACSM (2005).

guidelines for developing and improving muscular fitness are listed in table 2.4.

Adapting muscular fitness exercises for referred populations

As with other components of fitness, the intensity of activities selected should correspond to the following:

- the fitness level of the individual;
- the medical condition(s) with which they have been referred;
- the effects of any medication on the exercise response;
- any other specific lifestyle considerations (work etc.).

Previously inactive people will generally have to work at a lower intensity. They may also have lower levels of body awareness and muscular fitness and their exercise technique may demand more careful attention from the trainer (observation, correction, teaching) to enable safe participation. Fixed resistance machines provide more stability and support and may be more appropriate than free weights for referred clients beginning resistance training.

There are specific variants that can be altered to change and adapt the intensity of specific muscular fitness exercises. These are:

- resistance
- rate
- range of motion
- repetitions
- rest (between sets or exercises).

Resistance

There are numerous methods for altering the resistance. Muscular fitness activities can be progressed and adapted by:

- increasing (or decreasing) the length of the lever being moved (rear leg raise with bent leg or straight leg);
- adding body-weight to (or removing body-weight from) the end of the lever (curl-ups with hands on thighs or hands at side of head);
- working against gravity or working across gravity (push-ups against a wall or floor-based);
- adding an external resistance such as a fixed weight, free weight or exercise band (and altering the resistance);
- using water: water adds resistance to body movements and will alter the type of muscle contraction.

Rate and range of motion

Exercise should always be performed at a controlled speed to promote full range of motion of concentric and eccentric muscle work.

Varying the speed of an exercise will alter the intensity and may also change the focus on the muscle contraction. For example: varying the speed to work faster on the lifting phase and more slowly on the lowering phase will focus on the eccentric contraction range. Caution is advised when lengthening the eccentric phase, as this may cause delayed onset muscle soreness (ACSM 2005a).

It is generally recommended that muscle work be carried out through the full range of motion. However, there are some instances where isometric and static muscle work are more beneficial as a starting point, for example in training core stability and posture and for some joint mobility problems (osteoarthritis).

Repetitions, rest and sets

One set of 8–12 repetitions for all major muscle groups is the traditional guide for muscular fitness improvements for general populations;

however, the ACSM (2005) recommends a broader range of repetitions, i.e. 3–20. It is obvious that the number of repetitions and sets can be increased or decreased to meet different fitness goals (strength or endurance). The repetitions will also need to take account of any specific medical conditions the individual presents. For some individuals, as low as one repetition would be an appropriate starting point.

Motor fitness

Motor fitness is primarily a skill-related component of fitness and refers to a number of inter-relatable factors, which include:

- agility
- balance
- speed
- co-ordination
- reaction time
- power.

Benefits of motor fitness

Motor fitness requires the effective transmission and management of messages and responses between the central nervous system (the brain and spinal cord) and the peripheral nervous system (sensory and motor). The peripheral system collects information via the sensory system; the CNS receives and processes this information and sends an appropriate response via the motor system, which initiates the appropriate response.

Motor fitness can have an indirect effect on improving our ability to function in the other components of fitness. Development of specific skills can improve our performance of certain activities and enable more skilful movement and safer exercise techniques. This can help to reduce the risk of injury and will maximise both the safety and effectiveness of our performance. Managing our body-weight, manoeuvring our centre of gravity, co-ordinating our body movements, moving at different speeds, in different directions, and at different intensities, will all in the long term contribute to improving our motor fitness.

Guidelines for training motor fitness

Like all components of fitness, the principles of 'use it or lose it' and 'specificity' apply. What you train for is what improves, so running improves running and stretching the hamstrings makes more flexible hamstrings.

Older populations can sometimes lose the skilfulness of their movement, and therefore motor fitness will need to be retrained. Learning to balance and co-ordinate movement patterns takes time and it is essential to break the movement down into its simplest parts and progressively build on these. Relearning movement patterns also takes time. As a general guideline, starting more slowly, with isolated movements and simpler movement patterns, and focusing on correct performance, helps to provide the foundation for developing motor fitness. Patience, encouragement and raising awareness to small changes and progression are essential to maintain motivation.

TOTAL FITNESS AND LIFESTYLE

3

Total fitness

Total fitness provides a model for determining health and well-being. It requires balanced 'fitness' in all the following areas:

- **Physically** Achieving recommended levels of physical activity in daily lifestyle and taking part in exercise to maintain physical fitness: cardiovascular, muscular, flexibility and motor fitness as discussed in Chapter Two.
- **Socially** Being able to create and maintain healthy relationships with others and society.
- **Mentally** Having an awareness of personal thinking patterns and being able to manage thinking to assist positive decision-making and life choices.
- **Emotionally** Having an awareness of and the ability to manage and express emotions (happy, sad, scared, angry) assertively with respect for self and others.
- **Nutritionally** Eating a balanced diet containing a variety of foods from all major food groups (carbohydrates, fats, protein, vitamins, minerals, water, fibre), eaten within recommended guidelines, and maintaining a balanced calorific intake to meet energy demands.
- **Spiritually** Having an awareness of one's belief systems, which may evolve from family, society, culture and religion, and managing these to make positive decisions for self, others and society. Embracing the notion of difference and similarity among people.
- **Medically** Being free from illness and disease and making positive life choices to maintain medical health.

Total fitness requires a little bit more than just taking part in regular physical activity. It demands that we also pay attention to our lifestyle, diet, stress levels, emotions and ability to communicate, and recognise that sometimes it is important for us quite simply to relax and recuperate. Physical activity, exercise and physical fitness contribute to maintaining health and total fitness.

Social fitness

Social fitness relates to interaction and communication with other people and the ability to form and maintain healthy, functional relationships within society. Exercise and activity provide opportunities for social interaction and enable individuals to improve their social fitness.

Depressed clients in particular can feel very isolated and alone with the problems that contribute to their depression. In addition, the stigma attached to mental health conditions will influence how they feel about themselves and also how they perceive that others will think of them. It can be hard for them to motivate themselves to seek out a social network; however, the benefits are numerous.

Apart from the physical benefits of exercise and activity, group exercise in particular is an excellent medium for promoting social interaction and benefits. It naturally encourages networking and friendships to blossom among class members, and many additional social opportunities evolve from the relationships developed within the session. Since depression and other health conditions (osteoporosis, high blood pressure, arthritis etc.) are common to many people, support can be found in sharing experiences of how to manage the condition. It will also reduce feelings of being alone or the only person having to deal with the condition(s), which normalises the experience and can increase confidence towards participation in activity and self-management.

Mental and emotional fitness

Mental and emotional fitness refers to psychological well-being. The pressures of daily life can have a negative effect on our mental and emotional fitness, causing us to feel tired, anxious and stressed. The diagnosis of medical conditions (high blood pressure, osteoporosis, cancer etc.) will raise some degree of fear in most people regarding future mobility, independence, suffering and life expectancy.

When we feel stressed we stimulate the release of hormones that prepare us for fight or flight. As a consequence we release sugars into the bloodstream to provide energy for the necessary physical action. However, all too often we do not take action (fight or flight) and instead stew on our problems. This has a negative effect on our health because sugars are released, which can potentially contribute to atherosclerosis. Stress is therefore a contributory factor to a number of minor and major diseases, including: high blood pressure, coronary heart disease, irritable bowel syndrome and anxiety. It is wise to take some precautionary measures to reduce our stress levels.

As a method of managing stress, some people choose unhealthy habits such as the use of tobacco, alcohol, drugs, coffee or unsuitable food to help them manage emotions and provide a short-term fix for feeling better and coping. In the long term all these substances produce a negative effect and involve a further health risk. Information regarding support programmes to assist smoking cessation and management of drugs, alcohol and weight are available from most local primary care trusts, hospitals and GP surgeries.

Regular exercise and activity are excellent ways of managing the stress response. Physical exertion offers an excellent release for physical stress and the pressure and tension that build up in the muscles as a consequence of the stress response. It can also distract one from daily hassles or worries and help to clear the mind and assist thinking. Exercise promotes the circulation of endorphins, a compound of hormones that induce a feeling of well-being that can last for much longer than the duration of the activity. In addition, the longer-term benefits of exercise can all contribute to improved self-esteem, self-image and self-confidence.

Some group exercise sessions have a specific focus on relaxation and concentration. Pilates, yoga, tai chi and other mind and body style sessions all use specific techniques to focus the mind and enable meditation/relaxation techniques that can be used to assist with stress management and emotional well-being.

Nutritional fitness

Nutritional fitness requires us to eat a balanced diet of foods from all the major food groups in the appropriate quantities to maintain nutritional and energy requirements. The foods we eat will affect our energy levels and our health and well-being. There are no bad foods per se, just poor diets.

The main food groups are:

- carbohydrates (pasta, potatoes, bread)
- fats (cheese, milk, butter)
- proteins (grains, pulses, meat)

- vitamins and minerals (vegetables and fruit)
- water.

We should also ensure that the quantity of food we consume is appropriate to meet our energy requirements.

Taking part in regular physical activity can make us more aware of the food we eat and more conscious of our diet. There are many books devoted to nutrition; some of these are listed as references at the end of this book. Some general guidelines for improving our diet are:

- **Eat less saturated fat**: too much increases the risk of high cholesterol and furring of the artery walls.
- **Eat less sugar**: too much can cause tooth decay and contribute to overweight and obesity.
- **Eat less salt**: too much may elevate blood pressure.
- **Eat more complex carbohydrates**: too little will lower our energy levels.
- **Eat sufficient fibre**: too little may cause constipation and other bowel disorders.
- **Eat more fruit and vegetables** (five portions a day).
- **Eat a sufficient calorie intake**: too little will slow down our metabolism and make us feel lethargic; too much will make us put on weight and will be stored as body fat.
- **Drink more water**: too little fluid will cause dehydration and potential heat stroke and place an unnecessary stress on the heart.
- **Eat when you feel hungry**: if we do not eat when we feel hungry our blood sugar levels will be affected, causing us to overeat and/or eat the wrong type of foods to manage our sugar levels. In addition, some people confuse feeling hungry with other feelings/emotional experiences and can use food to bring comfort.

Eating more than we need for energy will contribute to overweight and obesity.

Spiritual fitness

The type of person we become and the choices we make can be influenced by belief systems, attitudes and values passed down through generations within families, schools, societies, cultures and religions. Each of these can impact our own belief systems and our mental outlook (how we view ourselves and our lives), emotional management (how we respond to our own feelings and emotions and to the feelings and emotions of others), our attitude to physical activity (our activity levels and whether we look at exercise as a pleasure or an inconvenience), our eating behaviour (the type of food we eat and the size of our plate), our lifestyle choices (transport, smoking, alcohol, hobbies) and our social relationships (how we relate to others, prejudices etc.).

From a spiritual perspective, each of us is a unique individual with our own life journey and our own life lessons. We each make choices to follow a different life path and we each have the potential to choose how we respond and grow from life's challenges and the events that contribute to the person we become. As Van Deurzen (2000: 333) suggests: 'some people manage to overcome substantial initial disadvantages or adversity, whereas others squander their advantage or flounder in the face of minor contretemps'.

Illness and experience of death (relatives, friends, world disasters) are particularly significant life events that can awaken the existential search to find answers for being, and can provide an opportunity for spiritual growth, which is a lifelong journey!

Spiritual fitness embraces the inner power we all have to love, create peace and live in harmony and balance within ourselves and in the world. Spiritual fitness recognises diversity and difference among people and introduces the possibility that people are all at different stages of growth. It embraces the notion that people make the right choices for themselves, with the knowledge and skills they have at a particular time, from which, together with their unique experiences, they can learn and grow as individuals.

From this perspective, we all have the power to make changes and make a difference in our own inner world, which impacts and contributes to our outer world.

Medical fitness

Medical fitness is our state of health; it requires the body to be in optimal working order. The evidence reported throughout Part Three indicates that medical fitness is declining among the population. Regular activity and keeping physically fit can reduce the risk of some diseases and contribute to the management of many of the medical conditions discussed in Part Three.

Regular exercise, activity and improved fitness can encourage us to eat a more nutritious diet, maintain a healthy body composition and manage stress more effectively. It can also build social networks and relationships, which in turn may encourage us to cut down or remove habits that have an adverse affect on our health, such as smoking, drinking too much alcohol or eating too many of the less nutritious foods, all of which contribute to an increasing risk to health.

Other lifestyle factors

Alcohol

The Department of Health 'Think about Drink' leaflet suggests that small, regular quantities acceptable alcohol are ok and can actually be beneficial for health, in that alcohol (in moderation) can offer protection against CHD by influencing blood cholesterol and reducing the likelihood of blood clots.

Drinking levels are measured by calculating the units of alcohol consumed on a daily basis. See the box below: 'Calculating the units of alcohol'.

Calculating the units of alcohol

Volume of millilitres multiplied by percentage alcohol by volume (% abv) divided by 1,000 = Number of units

Bottled beer:
330ml × 5 (% abv) = 1,650 divided by 1,000 = 1.7 units

Adapted from Department of Health 'Think about Drink' public information leaflet.

Too much alcohol can have detrimental effects on health. Drinking more than the recommmended levels/units of alcohol (see table 3.1) can increase the risk of liver damage, cirrhosis of the liver and cancer of the mouth and throat.

Table 3.1 Recommended daily units		
Units of alcohol and health risk	*Women*	*Men*
No significant health risks	2–3 units per day	3–4 units per day
Increasing risk to health	3 or more units per day on a regular basis	4 or more units per day on a regular basis

Table 3.2	Units of alcohol in popular drinks		
Half pint of average strength beer, cider, lager	Small glass of wine	Pub measure of spirits (vodka, gin, rum etc.)
(3.5% abv) 1 unit	(9% abv) 1 unit	(40% abv) 1 unit

Adapted from Department of Health 'Think about Drink' public information leaflet.

Alcohol is not recommended for certain medical conditions and/or medications that can be affected by alcohol, and caution may be advised.

Persons concerned about their drinking habits should seek professional help. Some information services are provided at the back of this book.

Stopping smoking

The negative consequences of cigarette smoking on health are well documented. Carbon monoxide and nicotine are the two chemicals in cigarettes that have the most impact on the heart. Carbon monoxide contributes to decreased oxygen being circulated around the body to the tissues. Nicotine stimulates the production of adrenaline, which increases heart rate and blood pressure, causing the heart to work harder. Smoking also damages the lining of the coronary arteries and contributes to atherosclerosis, a building-up of fatty tissue on the artery walls. The tar in cigarettes causes cancer.

Smoking is highly addictive and once started is not easy to quit. Persons who wish to stop smoking are advised to contact a local smoking cessation group to receive advice and support to help them quit. Some information services are provided at the back of this book.

Summary of the health and total fitness benefits of physical activity and exercise

Regular physical activity and exercise can:
- Maintain and improve mobility and flexibility
- Improve strength of bones and muscles
- Reduce the risk of osteoporosis
- Manage type 1 diabetes
- Prevent and manage type 2 diabetes
- Improve cholesterol levels
- Reduce the risk of high blood pressure, heart disease and stroke
- Assist with managing blood pressure
- Assist with weight management
- Promote social interaction
- Encourage a healthier lifestyle
- Improve sleep patterns and increase energy levels
- Assist with managing stress and depression
- Improve self-esteem and confidence
- Enhance feelings of well-being
- Prevent falls and injuries in older adults
- Manage joint and mobility conditions
- Improve posture and ease of movement
- Reduce the risk of certain cancers
- Improve ability to carry out everyday activities and help maintain independence
- Improve overall health

PLANNING TO WORK
WITH REFERRED CLIENTS

PART TWO

This section of the book discusses considerations for working with referred clients. It includes information on the referral process, screening, assessment, risk stratification, session structure and design, monitoring intensity and health and safety.

THE REFERRAL PROCESS, SCREENING, RISK STRATIFICATION AND ASSESSMENT 4

The Department of Health (2001a) sets out guidelines for the delivery of Exercise Referral in the National Quality Assurance Framework (NQAF) and offers specific guidelines for the pre-exercise assessment. This chapter discusses the referral process and assessment procedures.

The purpose of the referral and assessment process

A structured referral system, which includes a comprehensive client assessment, is essential to:

- assess the appropriateness of exercise/activity as an intervention for specific clients;
- develop a safe and effective exercise/activity programme;
- develop a programme that meets the needs of the individual, for example: cultural needs, social circumstances, exercise capacity, co-morbidities, preferences, etc.

The assessment process begins with the client's GP. This initial stage is the key to the referral procedure. For this stage to work effectively it is essential to establish the following:

- clear inclusion/exclusion criteria;
- well-designed and user-friendly paperwork;
- simple referral processes and procedures;
- named medical contact for each patient;
- effective working relationships;
- clear communication channels.

Clinical assessment

Before taking part in an exercise programme clients should be clinically assessed by their referring practitioner (GP). The NQAF (DoH 2001a) states that a referral form should include the following information:

- relevant current and past health problems;
- details of any medications being taken and their known impact on everyday functional ability;
- standard measures such as blood pressure (BP), heart rate, body mass index (BMI) and lifestyle factors, for example, smoking;
- the possible effects of diagnoses and medications on activities of daily living and, if known, exercise;
- any special considerations or advice given to the patient, for example: a patient with osteoarthritis should be advised to recognise and respect an increase in pain, stiffness or swelling;
- information about any exercise already being undertaken, or for which the patient or the referrer has expressed a preference, should also be included.

This information should be given in writing, using an exercise referral form. Information about a change in health status such as new symptoms or deterioration in an existing condition should also be communicated to the exercise professional (DoH 2001a). The patient should sign the referral form to agree to the transfer of this confidential information.

Medico-legal considerations

It is important for all parties involved in the referral process to be clear about the roles and responsibilities of all clinicians and others involved in the referral process and to maintain up-to-date knowledge of the medico-legal aspects. These are outlined in the NQAF (DoH 2001*a*). Table 4.1 summarises these roles and responsibilities.

The Medical Defence Union acknowledges the Register of Exercise Professionals (REPs) as a professional body, recognised by the Department of Health. GPs can refer patients to advanced fitness instructors (Level 3) with qualifications and experience of working with special/referred populations.

Informed consent

An informed consent should be obtained from the patient prior to undertaking the pre-exercise assessment and commencing an exercise programme (DoH 2001*a*). This provides an opportunity to discuss the proposed assessment and physical activity programme. An informed consent document should be written and provide the following:

* sufficient information, in accessible language;
* an explanation of the purpose of the exercise assessment and/or programme;
* a description of the components of the exercise assessment and/or programme;
* an explanation of the possible risks, discomforts and benefits;

* clarification of the responsibilities of the patient;
* a reference to confidentiality and privacy;
* an emphasis on the patient's voluntary participation and right to change their mind;
* the opportunity for the client/patient to ask questions (questions and answers can be recorded).

Informed consent is the client's agreement to participate in a pre-exercise assessment and exercise programme. It is not a legal waiver and if someone is not given sufficient information the document is not valid, even if it has been signed (DoH 2001*a*). Informed consent is part of an ongoing process, so any changes in an individual's health or exercise programme need to be discussed within the context of this document. Effective communication skills (see Part Four) are essential to the informed consent process to enable the client to feel comfortable to ask questions and clarify specific aspects of the assessment or programme.

Pre-exercise screening and assessment

The role of the exercise professional is to provide the appropriate support to enable the

Table 4.1	Roles and responsibilities
Role of the GP or referring clinician	*Role of the exercise professional*
Refer patient into a quality assured system.	Carry out pre-exercise assessment with the client.
Maintain clinical responsibility for the individual patient.	Refer back to the GP or referring clinician when appropriate.
Be responsible for the transfer of relevant, meaningful information to the exercise professional.	Be responsible for the safe and effective management, design and delivery of the exercise programme.
	Maintain patient confidentiality.

client to develop the skills, knowledge and confidence they need to become habitually more active. It is therefore important that they work in partnership with the client. Clients need to be actively involved in the process and in decisions regarding their health (DoH 2001*a*).

The pre-exercise screening and assessment process provides an opportunity to establish rapport with the client and gather information and take steps as follows:

- personal details (name, address, age, emergency contact);
- informed consent for the assessment process;
- relevant medical and health information including past medical history and current symptoms;
- medication (what type, how long taken for, any recent changes, effects on exercise);
- past and present activity levels, experience of physical activity;
- identify and discuss any misconceptions about exercise;
- assess client's exercise capacity using an appropriate assessment, e.g. walk test, step test;
- risk-stratify client using appropriate criteria;
- identify appropriate level of support and supervision;
- lifestyle information (work, habits, stress levels);
- expectations, goals, likes and dislikes (in relation to activity);
- readiness to change and self-efficacy and belief in their ability to make changes;
- personal motivation and desire to make changes;
- any positive strategies already in place (social support, counselling);
- any barriers that exist that may prevent them from making changes;
- mental attitude about their life and medical condition;
- any specific health needs that may require help of a specialist, such as a cardiac nurse or

physiotherapist (falls, stroke, cardiac event etc.);
- develop an appropriate exercise programme in partnership with client.

The structure and content of the pre-exercise screening and assessment will also depend on a number of factors including:

- transfer of appropriate information from GP (usually via the referral form);
- local protocols such as inclusion/exclusion criteria;
- resources such as time and appropriately qualified staff.

It is also important to consider the client's feelings and develop strategies to ensure the assessment has a positive impact on her or him. These considerations are discussed further in Chapter 14, Creating a Helping Relationship. Careful planning and preparation for the assessment offers the instructor the opportunity to:

- Provide the client with clear written information before s/he attends the session.
- Explain what will happen during the initial assessment, with clear instructions about what to wear and what to bring to the assessment.
- Prepare the environment to ensure that it meets health and safety requirements and is conducive to the assessment process. For example, images of older people walking and being active will be more appropriate than posters of young people in leotards and sportswear working out.
- Prepare for any special needs such as hearing loss or visual impairment.
- Ensure privacy and minimise interruptions.
- Make sure all the paperwork and equipment is available and accessible.
- Have relevant reference books available such as the British National Formulary (BNF).
- Use effective communication skills.

- Provide a non-judgemental and supportive environment.
- Adapt communication style to the needs of individuals, e.g. those with English as a second language.
- Find out about the client's expectations.
- Discuss client's concerns.
- Allow sufficient time to carry out the assessment in a meaningful way.

Using the information gathered during pre-exercise screening and assessment

It is important to go through the referral form with the client to confirm the medical information and discuss any changes in health since referral. It is also important to find out the client's perspective about his or her health. How informed are they about their health? How does their health affect their lives? Do they know about the role of exercise in relation to specific health conditions?

Screening and assessment information can be divided into the following sections

- demographics;
- reason for referral;
- current health status and past medical history;
- cardiovascular disease (CVD) risk factors;
- current medications and side effects/implications for exercise;
- psychosocial factors such as readiness to change, support network;
- exercise/physical activity history;
- personal goals.

1. Demographics (age, gender, ethnicity)

This information is collected for basic monitoring purposes. The relationship between age, gender, ethnicity and health is well established and it is important to consider these issues during the assessment process. For example, older people have an increased risk of cardiovascular disease, post-menopausal women have an increased risk of osteoporosis and South Asians living in the UK have a higher than average premature death rate from coronary heart disease (CHD) (British Heart Foundation 2005c).

2. Main reason for referral

This will usually be indicated on the referral form. There may be a mismatch between the GP's reason for the referral and the client's understanding of why s/he has been referred. This may provide an opportunity to find out more about the client's understanding about the referral and what his or her expectations are.

3. Current health status and medical history

This should include known diseases/conditions with dates (past and present), recent illness/surgery and current health status including blood pressure, resting heart rate and body-mass index (BMI). The quality of information provided on the GP referral form will influence the level of assessment the instructor carries out. For example, just knowing that someone has diabetes is insufficient. If someone with diabetes is referred, it is essential to know the date of onset, the presence of any diabetic complications, the client's experience of diabetes, how well managed the disease is and the last time the client had a hypoglycaemic episode.

If there are any new symptoms or changes to the client's health such as: new onset or worsening chest pain, orthopnoea (breathlessness that prevents individual from lying down), shortness of breath on exertion, claudication, palpitations, ankle swelling, dizziness or a recent fall, the instructor will need to refer the client back to the GP prior to exercise.

4. Cardiovascular disease risk factors

This information provides an idea of the person's CVD risk profile and ongoing lifestyle behaviours such as smoking and alcohol consumption. The person may be already be classified as at high risk of cardiovascular disease (CVD risk of ≥20 per cent over 10 years) by the GP. It may be useful to have a local health directory with information about services such as smoking cessation clinics, self-help groups and access to health promotion resources. When appropriate, this information can be given to clients to connect them with agencies that can provide more specialised support.

5. Medications and exercise implications

It is important to know what medications the client is taking because there are those that have implications for exercise. For example, beta-blockers suppress heart rate. The timing of medications may also be relevant for conditions such as diabetes or Parkinson's disease. If you have any concerns about the client's medication or feel the client needs more specific advice about it in relation to exercise, e.g. adjusting insulin dose prior to exercise, you will need to discuss this with the GP or refer the client back to the GP.

6. Social and psychological considerations

Social considerations The Health Education Authority (2000) identified a range of reasons specific to people from ethnic minority groups for not participating in physical activity. These included modesty, avoidance of mixed-sex activity and fear of going out alone. Other factors, such as fear of racism and socio-economic disadvantage, may also affect people's willingness to participate in physical activity in public places.

An isolated older person may prefer to attend a group session aimed at older people where the emphasis is on social support. They may prefer a daytime session, with easy transport links, at a time when they can use their free bus pass; however, this may not be the case and it is important not to make assumptions without checking first.

Psychological considerations An individual may be referred because of a mental health condition such as depression. Alternatively, s/he may be referred for another condition but also experience anxiety or depression. People with chronic health conditions such as asthma, chronic obstructive pulmonary disease (COPD), diabetes or arthritis often experience a range of emotions, including worries and fears about the future, frustration at not being able to do the things they used to do and feeling that they have lost control over their lives. These emotions are a common reaction to chronic illness and can lead to increased levels of anger and depression (NHS 2002). Some exercise referral schemes use questionnaires such as versions of the Short Form 36 (SF 36) or the Dartmouth COOP (a set of charts used to assess health status) to assess quality of life including feelings, social activities, pain, change in health and overall health and social support. This information can be used to identify people who may require specific support and to monitor changes over a period of time. It is important to use questionnaires that are valid and reliable for specific populations. Information about the SF 36 and the Dartmouth COOP are available from the Scottish Intercollegiate Guidelines Network (SIGN 2002).

Motivation and readiness to change are fundamental to long-term behaviour change and need to be central to the assessment process. This is discussed further in Chapter 15, Models of Behaviour Change.

7. Physical activity history

Previous levels of physical activity It is important to build up a picture of the client's experience of physical activity and/or exercise. The use of open questions can encourage the client to speak more freely and will enable the instructor to find out about what exercise means to the client, how important it is, and her or his personal experience of being sedentary or active. (Questioning skills are discussed further in Part Four.)

Current levels of physical activity
Measuring a client's physical activity level is an important part of the assessment process and it can be used in the following ways:

- to establish baseline activity level and monitor changes;
- to find out more about the client's current lifestyle;
- to facilitate discussion about the links between physical activity and the client's health;
- to educate the client about the frequency, intensity and type of activity beneficial for health;
- to identify barriers to physical activity;
- to facilitate behaviour change by developing appropriate interventions and support.

There are various subjective and objective methods that can be used to gather this information, including interviewer or self-administered questionnaires, e.g. seven-day recall, diaries and pedometers. The type of methods used will depend on a number of factors. These include:

- availability of local resources;
- the level of information required;
- the aim of the assessment, i.e. to get baseline information to help develop an appropriate exercise programme or to monitor changes over a period of time as part of an evaluation;
- motivation and co-operation of client;
- language and literacy skills.

The methods used will also need to be culturally appropriate and acceptable to the clients. Using more than one method will give you a more accurate picture of an individual's activity levels.

8. Personal goals

Identifying the individual's personal goals and developing a realistic plan can provide a framework in order to provide focus, motivation and a tool to review and monitor progress. If the client says s/he wants to be fitter, it is essential to try and find out what that means, by asking, for example: 'What sort of things do you want to be able to do? How will you feel?' It often helps to focus on behavioural goals as opposed to outcome goals, as these are easier to measure and monitor. Further information on goal-setting is provided in Part Four.

Screening and risk stratification

The ACSM (2005a) recommend different levels of screening to help with assessment and decision making. As a minimum a Physical Activity Readiness Questionnaire (PAR-Q) can be used as a basic screening tool prior to participation in an exercise assessment or programme. A commonly used screening tool is the Canadian PAR-Q developed by the Canadian Society for Exercise Physiology (2002). A physical activity readiness medical examination (PARmed-X), which consists of a physical activity-specific checklist, has also been developed for physicians to use with patients who have had positive responses to the Canadian PAR-Q. The Canadian PAR-Q is often adapted for use in UK exercise programmes.

Exercise contraindications

It is important for the referring GP to confirm that the patient exhibits no contraindications to exercise, such as:

- unstable angina;
- systolic blood pressure of more than 180mmHg and/or diastolic blood pressure of more than 100mmHg;
- BP drop >20 mmHg demonstrated during ETT (this will not be evident unless client undergoes an exercise stress test or has exercising blood pressure measured);
- resting tachycardia >100bpm;
- uncontrolled atrial or ventricular arrhythmias;
- unstable or acute heart failure;
- uncontrolled diabetes;
- febrile illness (such as flu or fever);
- acute systemic disease (such as cancers);
- neuromuscular, musculoskeletal or rheumatoid disorders that are exacerbated by exercise;
- unmanaged pain.

(Adapted from BACR 2005; ACSM 2005a.)

Risk stratification

The aim of risk stratification is to provide a safe and effective exercise programme at an acceptable level of risk, with appropriate monitoring and supervision. The main purpose of risk stratification is to identify and evaluate people who are at an increased risk of an exercise-related event specific to a disease process and provide appropriate monitoring and supervision. In the UK, most GP referral schemes have developed their own risk stratification tools, which identify people as high, medium or low risk. However, people do not necessarily fit neatly into categories. Risk stratification is important, but it needs to be used alongside clinical judgement and in conjunction with other activities such as client education and observation of the client during the exercise session. For example, a client who is stratified at high risk and well educated about her or his condition, is able to self-monitor and who complies with their exercise prescription is probably at less risk than a low-risk client who is unable to self-monitor and does not comply with the exercise prescription.

As well as focusing on the medical condition of the client it is important to look at the whole person; for example, the client's behaviour will influence the level of risk during exercise. The skills, knowledge, feelings and thoughts of the client will affect his or her behaviour and may influence the choice of exercise setting and the level of supervision required.

The ACSM (2005a) Risk Stratification Categories (see table 4.2) is designed for use once the following information is known:

- signs and symptoms of cardiovascular disease, pulmonary disease and/or metabolic disease;
- risk factors for coronary heart disease;
- known cardiovascular, pulmonary or metabolic disease.

Physical assessments

It is essential that the exercise professional is qualified and competent to carry out any physical assessments undertaken. It is important to consider both the reasons for conducting the assessment and the appropriateness of the assessment for the client. When conducting the assessment, the aims should be to involve the client as much as possible, provide clear explanations about the assessment and provide the client with the opportunity to ask questions.

Physical measurements

It is important that the exercise professional is qualified and competent to carry out any physical assessments. When conducting assessments, the

Table 4.2	ACSM Risk Stratification Categories
Low risk	Men <45 years of age and women <55 years of age who are asymptomatic and meet no more than one risk factor threshold (family history, smoking, hypertension, high cholesterol, impaired fasting glucose, obesity, sedentary lifestyle)
Moderate risk	Men ≥45 years and women ≥55 years or those who meet the threshold for two or more risk factors
High risk	Individuals with one or more of the following signs and symptoms: Anginal pain or discomfort Shortness of breath at rest or with mild exertion Dizziness or syncope Orthopnea or paroxysmal nocturnal dyspnoea (see note below) Ankle oedema Palpitations or tachycardia Intermittent claudication Known heart murmur or known cardiovascular, pulmonary or metabolic disease Cardiac (myocardial infarction, coronary artery bypass surgery, coronary angioplasty, angina) Cerebrovascular (stroke, transient ischaemic attack) Peripheral vascular disease Pulmonary disease (chronic obstructive pulmonary disease/cystic fibrosis, asthma) Metabolic disease (diabetes (Type 1 and Type 2), thyroid, renal or liver disease). Note: Othopnea refers to breathlessness (dyspnoea) occurring at rest in the recumbent position that is relieved by sitting upright. Paroxysmal nocturnal dyspnoea refers to breathlessness that usually begins 2–5 hours after going to sleep.

Refer to the ACSM's *Guidelines for Exercise Testing and Prescription* (2005) for detailed information.

aim should be to involve the client as much as possible and provide a clear explanation about what assessments are happening and their purpose and provide the client with the opportunity to ask questions.

Resting heart rate

Measuring a client's heart rate is a first step in checking whether s/he should take part in exercise. It can enable detection of:

- Normal heart rate 60–100 bpm
- Bradycardia (slow heart rate) <60 bpm
- Tachycardia (fast heart rate) >100 bpm
- An irregular heart rate.

A resting heart rate of >100 bpm is a contraindication for exercise and a client presenting this should be referred back to their GP. A client presenting with a slow resting heart rate should be assessed further to check whether they are on medication such as beta-blockers, which affect heart rate. A client presenting with a resting heart rate below 40 or who is experiencing symptoms such as dizziness should be advised not to exercise and referred back to their GP. (See Chapter 6, Health and Safety.)

Heart rate is affected by a number of factors which include:

- Medications
- Stress or anxiety
- Eating
- Smoking
- Caffeine
- Temperature.

Resting heart rate should be taken after the client has been sitting at rest for about five minutes. The most common site for feeling the pulse is the radial artery. It can also be felt at the carotid artery; however, it is essential not to press too hard at the latter point because pressure on the baroreceptors can cause a reflex slowing of the heart rate.

Most clients can be taught how to take their own resting heart rate. However, some clients may find this too difficult due to conditions such as diabetic neuropathy or obesity.

Resting blood pressure

This assessment provides the opportunity to identify:
- hypertension (i.e. persistent systolic blood pressure >140 mmHg and/or diastolic blood pressure >90 mmHg);
- hypotension (when blood pressure is lower than normal).

If the reading is higher than expected, the instructor should repeat the measurement at the end of the appointment. A systolic blood pressure of >180 mmHg and a diastolic blood pressure of >100 mmHg is a contraindication for exercise. Hypotension is usually asymptomatic; however, some people may feel dizzy or faint when they stand up. This is referred to as postural hypotension and may be caused by a number of conditions or the effects of medication such as beta-blockers or diuretics. The British Hypertension Society Guidelines (2004) recommend taking blood pressure in a standardised way, using a well-maintained, properly validated and calibrated device to ensure accurate and reliable measurements.

Body mass index (BMI)

BMI is used as a practical measure of fatness; however, it is not an accurate measurement for people who are very muscular or who have a very reduced muscle mass. Refer to Chapter 9, Obesity.

Waist circumference

Central obesity is associated with an increased risk of CHD and other cardiovascular disease. The easiest way to assess central obesity is by measuring the waist circumference. Refer to Chapter 9, Obesity.

Pulmonary function

Spirometry is the method used to measure lung function by measuring the forced vital capacity (FVC) and forced expiratory volume in 1 second (FEV1). The ratio of the two values is then calculated to give an indication of lung efficiency (YMCA 2004). FEV1 and FVC readings can be compared with normal values based on sex, age and height. Airflow obstruction is defined as:

- FEV1< 80% predicted, and
- FEV1/FVC <0.7

(BTS COPD Consortium 2005.)

Health professionals who have specific training normally carry out spirometry within Primary Care. Peak expiratory flow (PEF) is a more simple measure than FEV1, and repeat measures can be carried out at home using a hand-held peak flow meter. A normal peak flow is based on a person's age, height and sex and is expressed as a percentage of predicted peak expiratory flow. Clients usually work out a personal best with their GP and use that as a baseline for measurement. The pattern of peak flow measurement is just as important as the actual measurement. A peak flow meter provides a useful tool to support the self-management of asthma; however, it is not a sensitive measure for clients with chronic obstructive pulmonary disease (COPD).

Postural assessment

Posture refers to the alignment between various parts of the body. Optimal posture is important to minimise the stress placed on the body tissues and to ensure safe and effective exercise technique. Over a period of time poor posture may contribute to health problems such as tension headaches, joint problems and back pain. In clients with specific conditions such as Parkinson's disease or COPD, poor posture (kyphotis) can also lead to impaired respiratory function and postural instability. Posture can be assessed using a number of tools such as a standard reference line and a simple checklist to check the position of body parts such as shoulder blade alignment, level of skin creases and asymmetry in muscle bulk. Muscle imbalance contributing to poor posture can be addressed through re-education and strengthening of the postural muscles in conjunction with stretching exercises. Further information regarding postural assessment and improvement is discussed in other texts (Norris 2000).

Assessment of functional capacity

The Department of Health (2001 *a*) raises the issue of clinically testing referral patients in the National Quality Assurance Framework (NQAF). The Department of Health recognises that some patients may benefit from a medically supervised exercise test, while acknowledging that exercise testing is not financially viable and could act as a barrier to promotion of long-term physical activity. Clinical exercise testing is generally recommmended for higher-risk patients or individuals undertaking vigorous intensity exercise.

Clients of a low to moderate risk may be able to exercise at a moderate level of intensity without undergoing any specific assessment. Exercising at a moderate intensity minimises the risks associated with high-intensity activity and promotes adherence.

If an exercise assessment is to be included as part of the assessment process, it is essential to ensure that the assessment is individualised to meet the needs of the client, provides meaningful information and is a positive experience for her or him.

Pre-exercise assessments such as sub-maximal exercise tests can be useful to:

- educate the client about her/his current levels of fitness;
- collect baseline information that can be used to develop an exercise programme and tailor advice about activities of daily living;
- monitor progress and help motivate clients;
- assist risk stratification;
- gather useful information about a client's response to sub-maximal exercise including heart rate and rating of perceived exertion (RPE);
- explore difficulties the client has in terms of carrying out the assessment including following instructions, motor skills and the influence of co-morbidities.

(Adapted from Buckley and Jones, 2005.)

Key considerations for exercise assessments

- Think about what are you assessing and why. Do you want to find out about the client's aerobic fitness, endurance, muscular strength, flexibility, neuromuscular skills or functional performance?
- Ensure the test is appropriate to the needs of the client. For example, a 12-minute shuttle walk test (SWT) may not be appropriate for someone with Parkinson's disease who has difficulties initiating movement, turning and balancing, and a step test may not be appropriate for someone with an orthopaedic condition.
- Some clients may find the prospect of an exercise assessment anxiety provoking, which could be a barrier to exercise.
- If you perform a follow-up assessment, there may be a learning effect, which will influence the results.

Ongoing assessment and review

The process of pre-exercise screening and assessment can help to develop a strong foundation for encouraging long-term physical activity behaviour change. It will also enable a more structured exercise programme or exercise prescription to be developed.

However, the assessment process needs to be ongoing when working with referred clients. Before every session it is important to reassess the client's readiness to exercise and monitor any changes in health status. The assessment may include:

- any other changes in health from the initial assessment or previous session;
- response to previous exercise session such as excessive tiredness or discomfort;
- incidence of chest pain;
- the results/outcomes of any GP appointments and tests.

It can be helpful to plan regular review dates to assess progress, discuss any concerns that the client has and identify ongoing support needs. A structured one-to-one assessment provides the opportunity for the client to discuss any continuing concerns, such as, perhaps, their frustrations at not losing weight, or difficulties attending the sessions on a regular basis due to other responsibilities. Ongoing assessment enables the instructor to respond to the needs of the client, modify or progress the programme as appropriate and support concordance with their exercise programme.

EXERCISE PRESCRIPTION, MONITORING EXERCISE INTENSITY, SESSION STRUCTURE AND DESIGN

5

Exercise prescription

The aim of exercise prescription is to provide a safe and effective programme, reduce risk factors for chronic disease, increase fitness levels, promote overall health and encourage long-term behaviour change. Individual exercise prescriptions need to be based on the initial assessment process and take into account the following:

- current recommendations for specific conditions;
- FITT (frequency, intensity, time and type) principles to ensure a safe exercise programme with optimal rate of progression;
- health status;
- functional capacity;
- physical activity level;
- individual limitations, co-morbidity, risk stratification;
- interaction of medications and exercise;
- personal goals and preference;
- response to exercise (physiological and psychological);
- feedback from client.

A flexible and responsive approach to exercise prescription will ensure that the programme is adapted to meet the changing needs of the client, e.g. a client with Parkinson's disease may have daily fluctuations in their health status. Exercise prescription becomes increasingly complex with people with multiple co-morbidities and may require the input of a range of health professionals.

Progression of exercise

The initial goal is to engage the client in a regular exercise programme and rate of progression will be highly individual with any changes introduced conservatively, emphasising frequency and/or duration before intensity. Ongoing monitoring and feedback from the client will be important to ensure the progression is well tolerated, e.g. there is no increase in pain or tiredness. If there is a change in health status the client may be unable to exercise, e.g. if the client has a chest infection. When s/he returns to exercise the programme will need to be modified to take into account any loss of training adaptations due to inactivity.

Cardiovascular exercise intensity

The aim of setting cardiovascular exercise intensity is to ensure that the client exercises safely and effectively. If the intensity is too high, there is an increased risk of complications during exercise; if it is too low, the physiological adaptations associated with cardiovascular fitness will not occur. Ideally, exercise intensity should be based on the results of a functional capacity test carried out as part of the initial assessment, using a standardised step, cycle or walking protocol. These tests will provide baseline measurements such as heart rate, rating of perceived exertion (RPE) and estimated metabolic equivalents (METs), which can then be used to guide exercise intensity. See ACSM

(2005*a*) for detailed information on sub-maximal exercise tests.

In the absence of a functional assessment, you will have to base exercise intensity on subjective information about the individual's past and present levels of physical activity, along with their past medical history and current health status. You will need to start the client on a very conservative programme using heart rate, RPE, observation and client feedback to ensure an appropriate workload. Over a number of exercise sessions you can observe and record the client's response to specific workloads using different exercise modes, for example bike, treadmill or elliptical trainer, and use this as a baseline for developing the exercise programme. The methods most commonly used in the health and fitness setting for prescribing and monitoring cardiovascular exercise intensity include heart rate, rate of perceived exertion (RPE) and metabolic equivalents (METs).

Heart rate

Heart rate is widely used as a marker of exercise intensity. This is because of the linear relationship between heart rate and the oxygen demands of the muscles (VO_2) during sub-maximal exercise (ACSM 2005*b*). To calculate a target or training heart rate zone you need to know the maximal heart rate (HRmax); however, this requires an exercise stress test, which is impractical in a community setting. Alternatively, you can calculate HRmax based on the formula in the box above.

The age-adjusted HRmax should only be used as a guide as there is standard deviation (SD) of plus or minus 10-12 beats. This means that an individual may have an actual HRmax of 20 beats per minute higher or lower than the age-adjusted calculation, so relying on this formula to guide exercise intensity could potentially lead to an unsafe or less effective

Age-adjusted maximal heart rate (HRmax)

220 – age = age-adjusted HRmax

Example: Client (55 years old)

220 – 55 = 165

Adjusted for individual on beta-blockers

220 – age – 30 = age-adjusted-HRmax

Example: Client (55 years old)

220 – 55 – 30 = 135

exercise prescription. Medications such as beta-blockers can affect heart rate and this needs to be taken into account when calculating HRmax.

Methods for calculating target heart rate zone

The most common methods for calculating target heart rate range include:

- percentage of heart rate max (HRmax);
- karvonen method or heart rate reserve (HRR).

1. Percentage of maximal heart rate (%HRmax)

This method is based on the percentage of HRmax and is calculated using the actual or age-adjusted maximum heart rate. For example, if the target heart rate range is 60–75 per cent HRmax:

Step 1: Calculate age-adjusted HRmax
220 – age

Step 2: Calculate target heart rate range
HRmax × 0.6 = 60% HRmax
HRmax × 0.7.5 = 75% HRmaximum heart rate

2. Karvonen formula or heart rate reserve (HRR)

The Karvonen formula calculates the heart rate reserve (HRR) method to determine a target heart rate zone. The heart rate reserve is the difference between the HRmax and the resting heart rate and corresponds to the VO_2 reserve, e.g. 50–70 per cent HRR corresponds to 50–70 per cent of VO_2 reserve. VO_2 reserve is the difference between VO_2 max and resting VO_2. Where possible use an actual HRmax and an actual resting heart rate (ACSM 2005*b*).

To calculate 50–70 per cent HRR:

Step 1: Calculate HRR
HRmax (or age-adjusted HRmax) – resting heart rate = HRR
Step 2: Calculate training heart rate (e.g. 50–70% of HRR*)*
(HRR × 0.5) + RHR = 50% HRR
(HRR × 0.7) + RHR = 70% HRR

For example, Client X is 55 years old, his resting heart rate is 60 and his actual HRmax in unknown.

Monitoring heart rate response to exercise

It is difficult for people to take their own pulse during exercise and heart-rate monitors are recommended for pulse monitoring (SIGN 2002). Coded heart-rate monitors enable people to work in close proximity with other people wearing heart-rate monitors, without interference. Heart-rate monitors do not detect irregular heart-rates so it may be appropriate to use manual palpation with some clients. Heart-rate monitoring can be used alongside other methods of monitoring, such as RPE. Once clients are familiar with RPE and competent at using the scale they may not need to continue using a heart-rate monitor.

Method: % HRmax

To find 60–75% HRmax:

Step 1:
220 – 55 = 165

Step 2:
165 × 0.6 = 99
165 × 0.75 = 123.75

60–75% HRmax = 99–124

Method: HRR

To find 50 – 70% HRR:

Step 1:
220 – 55 = 165

Step 2:
165 – 60 = 105

Step 3:
105 × 0.5 = 52.5 + 60 = 112.50
105 × 0.7 = 73.5 + 60 = 133.50

50–70% HRR = 112–133

Rating of perceived exertion (RPE)

A perceived exertion scale can be used to quantify the subjective intensity of exercise (SIGN 2002). The participant is encouraged to focus on the sensations of physical exertion such as feelings of breathlessness, strain and fatigue in muscles and then to rate his or her overall feelings of exertion using a scale such as the Borg scale. The more experienced a client becomes at detecting and rating sensations, the more closely the ratings correlate with the exercise intensity. Borg developed two scales, the RPE 6–20 and the CR10 scales. The

Table 5.1	The Borg rating of perceived exertion (RPE) 6–20 Scale and the Borg category ratio scale (CR10)		
RPE Scale (overall sensations)		**CR10 Scale (individual sensations)**	
6	No exertion at all	0	Nothing at all	'No P'
7		0.3		
	Extremely light	0.5	Extremely weak	Just noticeable
8		1	Very weak	Light
9	Very light	1.5		
10		2	Weak	
11	Light	2.5		
12		3	Moderate	Strong
13	Somewhat hard	4		
14		5	Strong	
15	Hard (heavy)	6		
16		7	Very strong	
17	Very hard	8		
18		9	Extremely strong	'Max P'
19	Extremely hard	10		
20	Maximal exertion	11 •	Absolute maximum	Highest possible

P = perception
Adapted from Borg (1998).

6–20 scale (see table 5.1) is designed for rating overall feelings of exertion and is generally used for steady state aerobic activity, while the CR10 scale is designed for rating more individualised responses such as breathlessness and pain. The CR10 scale is more commonly used with clients with health conditions such as chronic obstructive pulmonary disease, where the rating of breathlessness is more relevant than overall feelings of exertion. Alternative rating scales are suggested for specific conditions such as angina and claudication (ACSM 2005*a*).

Guidelines for effective use of RPE scale

- Allow enough time to teach the scale to clients so it can be used as a safe and effective tool to monitor intensity.
- Measure RPE at varied work rates and using different exercise modes to confirm relationship between heart rate and workload.
- Ensure all staff are teaching and using RPE in a standardised way.
- Get client to anchor the lowest and highest level of exertion to known sensations.
- Encourage clients to practise using the scale outside the exercise environment.
- Use RPE throughout the session including the warm-up and cool-down.
- Use the scale when people are exercising, not between or after exercises.
- Ensure the RPE chart is clearly visible at each exercise.
- Encourage client to focus on sensations throughout the session.
- Be aware of factors which may influence RPE such as anxiety, depression, preconceptions of activity, activity mode, mood and distractions such as loud music.
- Ensure client can reliably estimate ratings of perceived exertion (estimation mode) before you hand the client the responsibility of self-regulating her or his exercise intensity (production mode).

Buckley et al. (1999).

Table 5.2 provides a useful classification of exercise intensities with corresponding description for, RPE, %HRR or VO_2R, and %HRmax.

Table 5.2	Classification of exercise intensity for cardio-respiratory endurance		
Intensity	*RPE*	*% HRR or VO_2R*	*% HRmax*
Very light	<10	<20	<35%
Light	10–11	20–39	35–54%
Moderate	12–13	40–59	55–69%
Hard	14–16	60–84	70–89%
Very hard	17–19	> 85	>90%
Maximal	20	100	100

ASCM (2005*b*).

METs (metabolic equivalents)

METs provide another method for guiding exercise intensity. One metabolic equivalent is defined as the amount of oxygen the body uses at rest:

1 MET = 3.5 ml of oxygen per kilogram of bodyweight per minute

METs are used to express the energy cost of physical activity as a multiple of the resting metabolic rate. During activity the oxygen demands increase to cope with the additional energy demands placed on the body. Activities are classified according to their oxygen requirements as multiples of the resting metabolic rate (1.0 MET). See table 5.3.

METs can be used to give advice about a range of activities, based on their known MET value, which the client can carry out within a safe exercise level. For example, if a client can walk at 3 mph (3.5 METs) at 70 per cent of their HRmax at 12–13 on the RPE 6–20 scale, one can prescribe a range of exercise equivalent to 3.5 METs and give people appropriate advice about activities of daily living and leisure activities.

Physical activity of <3 METS is classified as light intensity, 3–6 METS is moderate intensity and >6 METs is vigorous activity. For some

Table 5.3 Activities and metabolic equivalent (MET)	
Activity	MET
Washing face and hands	2.0
Light gardening	3.0
Walking at 2.5 mph (1 mile in 24 minutes)	3.0
Cycling (stationary bike, 50 watts, very light effort)	4.0
Walking at 3.5 mph (1 mile in 17 minutes)	4.0
Heavy gardening	4.0
Golf (walking and carrying clubs)	4.5
Cycling (stationary) 100 watts, light effort	5.5
Swimming leisurely	6.0
Walking at 4 mph (1 mile in 15 minutes)	6.0
Mowing lawn (hand mower)	6.0
Swimming (crawl, slow moderate or light effort)	8.0
Running 5 mph (12 min/mile)	8.0

Adapted from Ainsworth et al. (2000).

activities other factors such as environmental effect or individual technique will increase the MET value of an activity, e.g. windy weather or poor swimming technique. For further information about using METS to prescribe exercise, see ACSM (2005).

Monitoring exercise intensity

Effective monitoring of exercise intensity is a key safety factor in exercise. Exercising above a prescribed intensity level increases the likelihood of complications during exercise (AACPVPR 2004). It is important to educate clients about appropriate exercise intensity and teach then how to monitor exercise. Referring to the risks and benefits discussed within the informed consent can be a useful reminder for clients who do not adhere to their programme.

Monitoring resistance training

It is more difficult to determine appropriate intensities for resistance training. A common method for guiding intensity uses a percentage of 1 repetition maximum (1RM), which is the maximum weight that can be lifted once by a particular muscle group, e.g. 40–60 per cent of 1RM. Determining 1RM is impractical for referred clients and a conservative approach is more often used to find a weight that a client can lift comfortably for a set number of repetitions, e.g. 8–12. The ACSM (2005a) defines intensity as the effort required, or how difficult the exercise is. A resting muscle represents minimal effort and momentary muscular failure or fatigue in the concentric phase of contraction represents high intensity. For clients with high risk of cardiovascular disease or other chronic conditions, the ACSM (2005a) recommends stopping an exercise as the concentric phase of the exercise becomes

difficult (RPE 15–16), while maintaining good technique.

A low initial workload will reduce the risk of orthopaedic, musculoskeletal problems or elevated blood pressure response to training. The initial training period provides the opportunity to familiarise the client with resistance equipment and teach correct exercise technique with an emphasis on developing the client's competence and confidence in the safety of the exercise environment.

Observation

Observation is an equally important method for the instructor to assist detection of any changes in the client. Observation can be used to monitor:

* excessive breathlessness and changes in levels of breathlessness
* sweating
* pallor and changes in skin colour
* anxiety in relation to the exercise response
* loss of co-ordination and exercise technique.

Ideally, a combination of methods (heart-rate monitoring, RPE and observation) should be used to monitor exercise intensity.

Session structure

All sessions should include a warm-up, conditioning section and cool-down, and a comprehensive programme should include all the components of physical fitness. However, it may not be appropriate to target all components of fitness in every session. When working with referred populations, specific considerations and adaptations need to be made to accommodate the presented medical condition(s) and other factors that relate to the individual (age, medication, current fitness and activity levels). For some medical conditions it may be more appropriate to focus more specifically on a particular aspect of fitness, such as postural and functional movement for persons with back pain, or mobility activities to manage arthritis.

As a general guideline, with most referred populations the warm-up and cool-down components will need to be longer and of a lower intensity than for an apparently healthy individual and the main workout (cardiovascular and muscular fitness) will need to be tailored (intensity, type, duration) to accommodate the specific needs of the individual(s). Specific considerations are discussed in Part Three.

The warm-up

The aim of the warm-up is to prepare the body and mind for the activity to follow, to reduce the likelihood of injury or any adverse effects and to increase the effectiveness of the exercise session. A beneficial warm-up will increase body temperature, enabling the muscles to contract and relax more efficiently and the joints to move more freely. The warm-up also provides an opportunity to practise or rehearse movement patterns specific to the activity to follow, for example performing a pressing action with the arms in preparation for a wall press-up or chest press using resistance equipment.

Components of a warm-up

- **Pulse raising** which consists of low-level aerobic activity to warm the body and gradually raise heart rate. A gradual increase in intensity will decrease the likelihood of abnormal changes to heart rate and heart function.
- **Mobilising major joints** by taking them through a full range of movement, taking into account the range of movement required during the main workout.

- **Stretching major muscle groups** after active warm-up to elevate muscle temperature. Evidence about the role of stretching within the warm-up is inconclusive and you may want to consider the appropriateness of maintenance stretching or full-range mobility activities for your client within the warm-up.
- **Rehearsal of movement patterns,** specific to the activity to follow, to develop skill level and enhance performance.

As a general guideline, with most referred populations the warm-up and cool-down components will need to be longer and of a lower intensity than for an apparently healthy individual.

Main work-out or conditioning section

This section generally includes both cardiovascular and resistance training; however, with referred clients it may not be appropriate to include both fitness components within one session. For example, a client who has had a stroke may benefit from a focus on resistance and neuromuscular (e.g. balance and co-ordination) training in one session and cardiovascular training in a separate session.

Main considerations for referred clients

- Decide on use of interval approach v. continuous activity: clients with a limited exercise capacity may benefit from an interval approach with active rests.
- Select appropriate activity taking into account orthopaedic limitations, postural instability, etc.
- Choose level of impact, e.g. minimal impact for people with orthopaedic problems.
- Decide on level of support, e.g. when getting on or off equipment.

- Consider implications of medications, e.g. beta-blockers which suppress heart rate.
- Consider use of fixed machines and/or chair-based options if there are balance, stability or orthopaedic conditions.
- Floor-based activities may be inappropriate for some clients, e.g. those who are unable to get up and down without assistance, or have postural hypotension.
- Consider an emphasis on functional activities that will help clients perform activities of daily living (ADLs).

Refer to Chapter 2 (see pages 9–18) for adaptations for referred clients.

The cool-down

As with all exercise sessions, the cool-down needs to *return* the body physically and mentally to an appropriate pre-exercise state. A gradual reduction in exertion intensity is required to maintain adequate venous return and enable heart rate to return to near resting levels. Stretches to maintain and, where appropriate, develop flexibility can be included, along with breathing and relaxation exercises (see under 'Stress' in Chapter 7, pages 65–71). Referred populations may need to spend longer on the cool-down section. For example, older clients have an increased risk of blood pooling and also of hypotension (low blood pressure) following exercise. Specific considerations for medical conditions are provided in Part Three. With higher-risk clients a period of post-exercise observation may be important to ensure people are feeling well before they leave the exercise area. For many clients the post-exercise period provides the opportunity to develop social networks. This is especially important for people who may be socially isolated, such as older adults.

HEALTH AND SAFETY

6

When working with clients it is important to ensure a safe exercise environment. People who are suitably trained or who have the appropriate knowledge and skills can carry out risk assessment. There is usually someone within an organisation who is designated Health and Safety lead; however, it is the responsibility of all employees to identify risks and carry out appropriate action. A risk assessment involves identifying any significant risks or hazards present in the working environment or arising out of work activities.

Hazard A hazard is something that has the potential to cause harm; this could include faulty equipment, a slippery floor surface, teaching too many people in a confined space.

Risk A risk is the likelihood of potential harm arising from the hazard.

The Health and Safety Executive (2003) has produced a five-step guide which provides an introduction to carrying out a risk assessment in the exercise environment. The steps are outlined in table 6.1. Table 6.2 provides examples of hazards and control measures in the exercise environment.

The risk assessment must be tailored to the specific exercise environment, such as the client's home, a local park or a community venue. It is important to ensure your exercise environment is accessible to disabled people. Under the Disability Discrimination Act (1995), which aims to end discrimination against disabled people, and related legislation, service providers have a duty to give disabled people access to everyday services and to consider making reasonable adjustments to the way they deliver services so as to make that possible (Directgov, 2005).

Management of problems and emergencies in the exercise environment

Before every exercise session it is important to pre-screen clients to find out if there has been any recent change in health, including:

- change in symptoms, e.g. worsening symptoms of asthma, or onset of chest pain;
- new symptoms, e.g. pain in calf when walking;
- change in medications, e.g. beta-blockers, insulin;
- the results of any tests or investigations;
- exacerbation of existing joint problems;
- new joint problems, e.g. knee or back problems;
- feeling unwell, e.g. sore throat or cold;
- any other health-related concerns, e.g. increasing fatigue, low mood, depression.

The pre-exercise assessment is an important aspect of minimising risk and reducing the likelihood of adverse incidents during exercise. It also provides the opportunity for ongoing client education, for example reminding clients to check blood glucose levels. The information gathered can be used to inform decision making about exercise participation and provide an appropriate intervention. These decisions may include:

- postponing exercise until client feels better, e.g. after cold or sore throat;
- referring back to GP for reassessment;
- modifying exercise session, e.g. avoiding upper-body resistance exercise if there are problems with a shoulder joint;

Table 6.1	Risk assessment
Step 1	**Identify the hazard** Concentrate on significant hazards Ask other people involved in the activity Use own knowledge and experience
Step 2	**Who might be harmed?** e.g. exercise professional, clients, carers
Step 3	**Evaluate risk** To evaluate the risk you need to consider: the likelihood of the harm occurring, the potential severity of the harm, and the people who might be exposed to the harm. Risk is often classified as high, medium or low. The risk may change depending on the person involved; for example, the risk of an older person with poor co-ordination and balance falling off a treadmill is higher than for a younger person with good co-ordination and balance. Safeguards need to be in place to control the risk so that harm is unlikely. You then need to decide whether you have done enough to minimise or control the risk or whether you need to take further precautions. Some hazards may require additional assessment, e.g. lifting, moving and handling.
Step 4	**Record your findings** Record hazards and the controls that are in place to minimise the risks
Step 5	**Review and revise** Set a review date. If there are any changes to working practice, e.g. new equipment, changes of venue, or different client groups, the risk assessment may need to be amended.

Adapted from *Five Steps to Risk Assessment* (HSE 2003).

- exercising with increased level of monitoring, e.g. if a client has slightly elevated blood glucose levels and is asymptomatic, it may be appropriate to advise him or her to begin exercise, then monitor blood glucose levels to check response.

Clients with any symptoms or conditions that are contraindicated, should not be allowed to exercise until they are resolved (see Chapter 4).

If a deterioration in the client's functional capacity is noticed, this should prompt the instructor to ask further questions about other factors, such as concordance with their home-based exercise programme or medication. If there is no apparent reason for the deterioration in functional capacity, the client should be referred back to her or his GP. A standard GP letter indicating clear reasons for referral can facilitate this process. Before a client can resume exercise, confirmation from the GP that it is appropriate for the client to continue with a structured exercise programme is required. The client's consent is required when additional medical information is requested from GPs. These issues are discussed in Chapter 4, The Referral Process.

It is important to document any changes in health, including type of symptoms, any change in pattern or relevant factors in client notes,

Table 6.2	Examples of hazards and control measures in the exercise environment
Hazard	**Control measures**
Equipment Injury associated with faulty equipment or inappropriate use of equipment	Exercise instructor to check that equipment is in good working order, and set up correctly. Carry out regular maintenance/calibration of equipment. Carry out appropriate induction, tailored to meet the needs of the client. Provide appropriate level of supervision.
Confined space Collision with equipment or other people	Ensure adequate space for activity and number of clients. Use effective teaching techniques to ensure client safety.
Slips, trips and falls Injury as a result of a fall	Check area is safe for use, e.g. no spillages, trailing leads, slippery floors. Ensure area is dry and safe after any mopping of area. Advise clients about appropriate footwear and clothing. Assess clients to identify individuals at risk of falling. Adapt exercise to meet the needs of clients, e.g. speed, transition, step patterns, equipment used.
Temperature e.g. dehydration	Check temperature. Adapt or postpone exercise. Ensure drinking water is available.
Fire	Check that emergency exits are clear and unlocked. Point out exit doors and fire points prior to session. Ensure adequate staff training.
Exercise-induced complications e.g. hypotension, hypoglycaemia, angina, cardiac arrest	Staff must be appropriately qualified. Clients should be assessed and risk-stratified. Clear inclusion/exclusion criteria must be in place. Exercise programmes are to be individualised according to risk stratification and individual limitations. Maintain up-to-date client information. Provide appropriate client education, e.g. how to monitor exercise intensity, recognise signs and symptoms of angina, etc. Pre-screen participants prior to each exercise session. Maintain an appropriate level of supervision and observation. Provide regular basic life support training. Ensure protocols are in place for the management of incidents and medical emergencies during the exercise session. Provide ready access to first aid personnel and equipment. Provide ready access to a telephone.

along with any action taken. An incident or accident book should be used to report any adverse events.

In spite of carrying out a risk assessment and pre-screening clients before exercise, there is always the potential for the development of complications before, during and after exercise. An action plan outlining the main problems likely to be encountered provides a useful framework for managing medical problems and emergencies within the exercise setting. The action plan in Table 6.3 gives some examples of medical problems which may occur along with appropriate actions. Action plans need to be developed in line with local protocols and will be informed by the exercise setting and level of staff training, e.g. whether staff are trained in the use of automated external defibrillators (AEDs). Follow-up procedures might include:

- reporting of incident/accident in line with local protocols;
- updating of client records;
- review of procedures and risk assessment;
- dissemination of any changes to procedures or risk assessment to other team members;
- debriefing – the opportunity to discuss any feelings associated with the incident;
- reassessment of client and review of exercise programme if appropriate.

Table 6.3	Management of problems and emergencies in the exercise environment

After any problem or emergency, follow reporting procedure, update client records and, if appropriate, review risk assessment.

Event/problem	Signs and symptoms	Immediate action	Further action
Angina	Pain in the chest, arm, throat, neck, back, shortness of breath. (In some cases people have non-typical pain or there may be no symptoms at all.)	• Client to stop exercising and sit down. • Assess client. • If client uses GTN advise to take 2 puffs spray or 1 tablet GTN. • Repeat at 5-min intervals up to 3 doses. • If pain relieved after one or two doses, wait 5 minutes. If appropriate, resume exercise at lower intensity. • If the symptoms of angina continue after third dose of GTN call 999 and inform of suspected MI. If angina is different or more severe than usual call 999 and inform of suspected MI. • Monitor client and respond to any changes. • Reassure client.	Refer to GP re: symptom control. Liaise with GP.

Table 6.3	Management of problems and emergencies in the exercise environment cont.		

After any problem or emergency, follow reporting procedure, update client records and, if appropriate, review risk assessment.

Event/problem	Signs and symptoms	Immediate action	Further action
Angina cont.		• Reassure other class members. • Provide paramedics with relevant information. • Contact relative/emergency contact. • If pain relieved after 15 minutes remain with client while they rest. Do not resume exercise. Arrange escort home if appropriate.	Refer to GP.
Change in pattern of angina In pre-exercise assessment client reports a change in pattern of angina since last exercising	Including: • worsening angina • angina on minimal exertion • angina at rest • sudden severe chest pain at rest	• Do not exercise. This may indicate unstable angina, which is a contraindication for exercise. If left untreated unstable angina may lead to a myocardial infarction. Ask client to see their GP soon. • Advise client to call 999 if they experience sudden severe chest pain at rest.	Refer to GP.
Myocardial infarction (MI)	Pain in chest, radiating to arm, throat, neck and back. Prolonged, severe pain, not relieved by GTN. Pallor, sweating, nausea, vomiting, dizziness. (Clients may experience severe symptoms, have mild chest pain or generally feel unwell.)	• Assess client. • Call 999 and inform them of suspected MI. • Ask client to adopt a half-sitting position with head and shoulders supported and knees bent (W position). • Encourage client to take their medication for angina. • Monitor client and respond to any changes in condition. • Reassure client. • Reassure other class members. • Provide paramedics with relevant information. • Contact relative/emergency contact.	Liaise with GP.

Table 6.3	Management of problems and emergencies in the exercise environment cont.		

After any problem or emergency, follow reporting procedure, update client records and, if appropriate, review risk assessment.

Event/problem	Signs and symptoms	Immediate action	Further action
Cardiac arrest	Absence of pulse and respiration.	• Call 999. • Commence basic life support (BLS). • Reassure other class members. • Provide paramedics with relevant information. • Contact relative/emergency contact.	Liaise with GP.
Collapse	A sudden faint or loss of consciousness. Pallor, sweating, rapid pulse.	• Assess client (consider diabetes, epilepsy or hypotension). • If unconscious, breathing and with a pulse, place in recovery position and call 999. • Monitor client and respond to any changes in condition. • Reassure other class members. • Provide paramedics with relevant information. • Contact relative/emergency contact. • If client regains consciousness consider GP or 999 as appropriate.	Liaise with GP regarding cause of collapse.
Arrhythmias Tachycardia	Heart rate >100 bpm	• Assess client and check BP. • If new onset or client is symptomatic refer to GP or call 999 as appropriate. Check for any change in medication.	Refer to GP.
Bradycardia	Heart rate <60 bpm	• Assess patient and check BP. • Check whether client is on beta-blocker. • If asymptomatic client can exercise unless <40 bpm.	Refer to GP.
Irregularity		• Assess client. • Check BP. • Check whether new onset. If symptomatic, e.g. feels faint, dizzy or lethargic, refer to GP or call 999 as appropriate.	Refer to GP if new onset.

Table 6.3	Management of problems and emergencies in the exercise environment cont.		

After any problem or emergency, follow reporting procedure, update client records and, if appropriate, review risk assessment.

Event/problem	Signs and symptoms	Immediate action	Further action
Arrhythmias Irregularity cont.		• Monitor and reassure client. • Provide paramedics with relevant information. • If treated and client is asymptomatic monitor weekly.	
Hypotension	Dizziness, fainting	• Assess client. • Check BP and heart rate. • Lie client flat and elevate feet. • Check for any change in medications. • Ensure recovery before travelling home and arrange escort home if appropriate.	Refer to GP.
Hypertension	Usually no symptoms, however may be detected on BP check	• If BP unusually high for individual recheck after resting for 5 minutes. If still higher than usual modify exercise programme and monitor. • Do not exercise if systolic >180 mmHg and diastolic >100 mmHg • Discuss concordance with medication.	Write to GP. Refer to GP.
Hyperglycaemia Hyperglycaemia is more likely to occur in individuals who take insulin. In adults symptoms usually develop over 1–2 days.	Blood glucose levels >13 mmo/l before exercise. Confusion, nausea, headache, thirst, abdominal pain, vomiting, hyperventilation	• Do not exercise if signs and symptoms of hyperglycaemia or if blood glucose levels >13 mmo/l and rising. If appropriate, test for ketones. If ketones are elevated do not exercise, due to increased risk of diabetic ketoacidosis. Advise client to contact healthcare team immediately to discuss appropriate action or call 999 as appropriate. • If unconscious, breathing and with a pulse, place in the recovery position and call 999. • Monitor client and respond to any changes in condition.	Refer to GP/diabetes healthcare team. Liaise with GP.

Table 6.3	Management of problems and emergencies in the exercise environment cont.		

After any problem or emergency, follow reporting procedure, update client records and, if appropriate, review risk assessment.

Event/problem	Signs and symptoms	Immediate action	Further action
Hyperglycaemia cont.		• Reassure other class members. • Provide paramedics with relevant information. • Contact relative/emergency contact.	
Hypoglycaemia (Clients with Type 2 diabetes who are not on insulin or hypoglycaemic agents are very unlikely to have a hypo.)	Blood glucose levels: <4.00 mmo/l before exercise or a sudden drop in blood glucose levels. 5–6 mmo/l before exercise During exercise: palpitations, muscle tremors, confusion, unreasonable behaviour, coldness, clammy skin, sweating, pallor, weakness, fainting or hunger, tingling lips. Deteriorating level of response.	• Do not exercise • Consume sugary snack (10–15 g) for light to moderate exercise and ensure blood glucose levels rise before commencing exercise. Increase intake according to the intensity and duration of the activity. • Stop exercise and sit client down. • Give sugar, e.g. a glass of fruit juice, not diet drink; three glucose sweets; followed by a starchy snack such as a sandwich, biscuits or bowl of cereal. • If unconscious, breathing and with a pulse, place in recovery position and call 999. • Monitor client and respond to any changes. • Reassure other class members. • Provide paramedics with relevant information. • Contact relative/emergency contact.	Refer to GP/diabetes healthcare team.
Asthma	Client needs to use inhaler more than once a day, is having difficulty sleeping or their peak flow reading has fallen below normal.	• Do not allow client to exercise, as asthma control needs to be improved.	Refer to GP to discuss asthma control/check inhaler technique.

Table 6.3	Management of problems and emergencies in the exercise environment cont.

After any problem or emergency, follow reporting procedure, update client records and, if appropriate, review risk assessment.

Event/problem	Signs and symptoms	Immediate action	Further action
Asthma cont.	Wheeze, cough, chest, tightness, shortness of breath	• Encourage client to take 2 puffs or more of reliever straight away, preferably using a spacer. • Encourage client to keep as calm as relaxed as possible. • Client should sit down and rest hands on knees for support. • Encourage client to slow down breathing to conserve energy. • Wait 5–10 minutes. • Do not resume exercise.	As above.
	Life-threatening symptoms: The reliever medicine is having no effect on symptoms Client too breathless to talk or eat, too tired to breathe normally, confused or irritable, looking pale or blue in colour	• If the reliever has no effect and/or client has life-threatening symptoms, call an ambulance. • Encourage client to continue using reliever every few minutes until help arrives. • Monitor client and respond to any changes. • Reassure other class members. • Provide paramedics with relevant information. • Contact relative/emergency contact.	Liaise with GP.
COPD	Excessive breathlessness People with COPD may have an increased risk of CHD; it is therefore important to be aware of symptoms of angina during exercise. (See section on angina)	• Encourage client to stop, adopt a comfortable position, either seated or standing, and allow breathing to return to normal. • Use inhaled medication as appropriate.	Refer to GP if symptoms worsen.
Stroke	Facial weakness, drooping mouth or eye Arm weakness, inability to raise both arms	• Stop exercise immediately. • Sit client down. • Call 999 and inform of suspected stroke.	Liaise with GP.

Table 6.3	Management of problems and emergencies in the exercise environment cont.		

After any problem or emergency, follow reporting procedure, update client records and, if appropriate, review risk assessment.

Event/problem	Signs and symptoms	Immediate action	Further action
Stroke cont.	Speech problems, inability to speak clearly or understand what you say	• Reassure client and monitor. • Provide paramedics with relevant information. • Contact relative/emergency contact.	
TIA (Transient ischaemic attack)	Symptoms same as stroke but effects last 24 hours or less and may pass within a few minutes.	• Stop exercise immediately. • Treat as a medical emergency even if symptoms subside after a few moments. Treat as suspected stroke, as above.	Liaise with GP.
Accident or incident		• Ensure safety of both casualty and other participants. • Monitor client as appropriate • Access appropriate services.	

(BACR 2000; Asthma UK 2005; Diabetes UK 2003*b* and 2004*a*; Stroke Association 2005*d*)

MEDICAL CONDITIONS, MEDICATION AND EXERCISE GUIDELINES

PART THREE

This section of the book discusses specific medical conditions and the exercise guidelines and considerations for working with persons with these medical conditions. It should be noted that most referred clients present with a combination of conditions and therefore the guidelines and considerations in relation to each condition need to explored and adapted to work with the specific individual, with guidance from and collaboration with the referring health professional.

MENTAL HEALTH CONDITIONS

7

There is no clear, single boundary that creates a defining point between what is considered mental health and what is considered mental ill-health or illness. An individual's classified mental well-being probably teeters somewhere along a continuum between the polar extremes of what psychiatric experts might refer to as functional (healthy) and dysfunctional (not healthy) thinking, perception, responding, behaving, personality, intellect and emotion; i.e. those aspects of functioning that are not specific to a bodily system, unlike, for instance, gastro-intestinal and respiratory functioning (Daines et al. 1997). A psychiatrist generally uses the term 'mental illness' when there is a clear range of signs and symptoms (referred to as a syndrome) present and where there is a distinct deterioration in the person's functioning (Daines et al. 1997). Some of the factors that contribute to the controversy of defining where the cut-off point is are introduced below.

Social and cultural factors: A person's behaviour and response to specific life events and circumstances is highly impacted by the cultural and social group to which s/he belongs. What is considered normal by one culture or social group (including families) can often be seen as abnormal by another culture and social group. With this in mind, it is suggested that the notion of similarity and difference between different groups needs to be explored and embraced before any classification is made regarding what is considered 'normal'. Persons interested in reading further in this area are referred to the ideas and viewpoints expressed by Fernando (1988), Gross and McIlveen

(1998: 562–613), Lago and Thompson (2003), Mindell (1995) and Rack (1982).

Stereotyping/labelling: Being classified as having a mental illness tends to create a stigma, which contributes towards stereotypical views towards such a person being adopted. These views can lead to separation and exclusion. Classifying a person as having a specific mental condition is intended as a guide and starting point to assist their treatment planning. However, there appears to be a general fear, discomfort and ignorance concerning persons with mental and emotional distress. This is compounded by the media's tendency to link mental illness with criminal violence. Spearing (1999) suggests, in particular, that persons with schizophrenia are not prone to violence; with the exception of those persons who have a criminal record before becoming ill or those with substance and alcohol abuse problems. She continues that 'most violent crimes are not committed by persons with schizophrenia and most people with schizophrenia do not commit violent crimes'. She also suggests that: 'substance abuse significantly raises the rate of violence in people with schizophrenia but also in people who do not have any mental illness'. With this in mind, it is suggested that stereotyping is not helpful as it can contribute towards impeding a person's recovery. Stereotyping in itself can be viewed as 'pathological' (Gross and McIlveen 1998: 456). The Mental Health Foundation (2000) suggests that the stereotypes portrayed are often 'contradicted by ordinary people's experiences of mental health problems affecting themselves, their family members, friends or work colleagues'. See also Daines et al. (1997).

Classification: Each of the major models that contribute to the study of human psychology and behaviour: *medical, biological, psychodynamic, behavioural, cognitive, humanistic* and *social*, have their own theories regarding how mental, emotional and behavioural disturbances can occur and how they should be treated. The most influential model has been the medical model, which identifies collections of signs and symptoms (a syndrome) that lead to diagnosis of specific mental conditions against the classificatory systems (ICD-10 and DSM-IV). These models imply that mental health problems are primarily caused by biological and medical factors; hence, treatment plans tend to rely heavily on medication. An introduction and overview of the classificatory systems is provided in Gross and McIlveen (1998). As the Mental Health Foundation (2000) suggests, 'most mental health problems result from a complex interaction of biological, social and personal factors'. With this in mind, while diagnosis of a specific condition can guide the planning of medical treatment, other contributory factors, such as social support systems, impact of stressful life events, etc. should also be considered for guiding treatment plans. As Daines et al. (1997: 68) suggest, 'no single model can provide all the answers, so an experienced psychiatrist learns the value of eclecticism of working as part of a team' within both primary care (GP, practice nurse, counsellor) and secondary care (psychologist, social worker).

This chapter introduces and describes some of the main mental health conditions classified and proposes a range of interventions that can be used for their treatment. Specific exercise prescriptions are comparatively limited and are left open to interpretation, as the severity of the diagnosed condition, prevalence of other medical conditions and prescribed medications will impact the exercise and/or activity intervention. These need to be taken into consideration by exercise professionals working with this population.

Depression

Depressive disorders are conditions that embrace a wide range of signs and symptoms that adversely impact the body (physical and behavioural), thinking (mental) and mood (emotional). It is not the same as a passing low mood, as it can cause more serious problems that impact daily living (how a person eats, sleeps, thinks and feels about themselves and the world and how they cope) and in severe instances it can lead to suicide. Of all the psychological disorders, it is the one that is most commonly seen by GPs. The World Health Organisation ranks depression as one of the leading causes of years lived with a disability worldwide, and places it second only to ischaemic heart disease in developed countries.

Major depression is diagnosed when a there are a number of symptoms present that interfere with daily functioning (work, sleep, eating and ability to enjoy activities and hobbies that were previously pleasurable) and these are accompanied by a low mood for a minimum of two weeks. A major depressive episode can occur only once but more frequently occurs more than once during the lifespan. Without treatment, the symptoms can last for months or years (Strock 2000).

Bipolar disorder or manic depression is less prevalent than other types of depression and is characterised by extreme mood swings that range from euphoria (manic phase) to severe lows (depressive phase). Diagnosis involves the experience of one or more manic/mixed episodes accompanied by a major depressive episode.

Cyclothymia and dysthymia The symptoms for these conditions are less disabling or severe and therefore do not warrant the diagnosis of a major depression; however, they will still prevent a person from feeling good about him- or herself, and may affect some functioning; but there is no drive to commit suicide. The symptoms also need to be experienced for a longer period of time, a period of approximately two years (Davison and Neale, 2001). Cyclothymia combines symptoms of mania and depression. Dysthymia is non-episodic chronic depression.

Causes

There are various theories regarding the causes of depression:

- biological (brain chemistry);
- genetic disposition (heredity);
- environmental and social factors (stress, relationship problems, illness, bereavement, loss of job, life transitions, etc.);
- psychoanalytic (early developmental experiences);
- cognitive-behavioural (thinking patterns);
- humanistic (low self-worth);
- family systems (relationships and roles within the family).

As Strock (2000) suggests, a combination of these factors can contribute to onset of the condition and later episodes may be 'precipitated by only mild stresses, or none at all'.

Prevalence

According to the Mental Health Foundation, 'One in four women and one in ten men will experience an episode of depression serious enough to require treatment at some point in their life' (Halliwell 2005: 13). Therefore, the ratio of women to men experiencing depression is 2:1 (Strock 2000). This may be due to hormonal factors that affect women (menstruation, pregnancy, birth, etc.) and/or other responsibilities (caring for children and/or elderly relatives, work). Alternatively, Strock (2000) suggests that depression in men may be 'masked by alcohol and drugs' and that men are less likely to admit to feeling depressed. She also suggests that depression in men tends to be displayed as irritability and anger and that men may be less inclined to ask for help.

It is estimated that over 20 per cent of individuals with major depression never seek help nor are seen by their GP and that 40 per cent of those with depression are not recognised by their GP because they present with another, physical, illness (Daines et al. 1997). It is further estimated that mild to moderate depression affects over 7 per cent of adults at any one time. Approximately 15 per cent of severely depressed adults commit suicide after only one month of a first episode.

Signs and symptoms

Emotional Persistent sad, anxious or empty mood, feelings of hopelessness, pessimism, guilt, worthlessness, helplessness, irritability, inability to express or experience pleasure in previously enjoyed activities (Strock 2000; Davison and Neale 2001).

Mental Negative outlook on life, self and environment, suicidal thoughts (with or without intent), inability to focus and concentrate, or make decisions (Strock 2000; Davison and Neale 2001).

Behavioural Changes in appetite (over- or under-eating) and/or libido, deterioration in relationships, withdrawal from supportive relationships, increased smoking and/or use of alcohol, change in work or academic performance (Strock 2000; Davison and Neale 2001).

Physical Decreased energy, motivation, lethargy, changes to sleep patterns (insomnia or oversleeping), fatigue, weight loss or gain (contributed to by changes in eating patterns), persistent physical symptoms that do not respond to treatment (headaches, aches and pains, gastroenteritis), which mask the psychological symptoms (Strock 2000; Davison and Neale 2001).

Bipolar disorder (manic depression)

Persons experiencing bipolar disorder will display a range of signs and symptoms from extreme lows (during the depressive phase) to extreme highs (during the manic phase).

Depressive phase Some of the signs and symptoms suggested above for major depression.

Manic phase Abnormal or excessive euphoria/elation, decreased need for sleep, increased libido, grandiose notions, increased energy, irritability, rash and inappropriate social behaviour, racing thoughts and speech (Strock 2000; Davison and Neale 2001).

Treatment

There are numerous treatments for depression, depending on the severity of the diagnosis. They range through conventional drug therapy, ECT and psychological and counselling therapy. Other alternative treatments, such as

homeopathy etc., may be used alongside or instead of orthodox medicine. More recently, the Mental Health Foundation has introduced the 'UP and Running' campaign which cites the benefits of exercise and some specific research to promote exercise as part of the treatment programme for persons with mild to moderate depression (Halliwell 2005).

Medication

A variety of drugs can be used in the treatment of depression. Some of these are listed at the end of this chapter.

Antidepressants These are the most commonly prescribed drugs to treat depression. In particular, SSRIs (selective serotonin reuptake inhibitors) are prescribed as they have fewer side effects than other medications. They affect neurotransmitters (dopamine and norpinephrine). MAOIs (monoamine oxidase inhibitors) and tricyclic antidepressants are used less frequently because of adverse interactions with other drugs and more frequent side effects. Antidepressants help to reduce the symptoms of depression and boost motivation (Strock 2000).

Anti-anxiety drugs or sedatives These are sometimes prescribed alongside antidepressants to assist with anxiety and promote sleeping. They are not effective for treating a depressive disorder if taken alone (Strock 2000). The most commonly used is the benzodiazepine (BDZ) group. They produce effective short-term benefits but are highly addictive and therefore not recommended for long-term use.

Mood-stabilising drugs These are used to treat severe depression and bipolar disorder by stabilising the mood. The most common is lithium.

Anti-psychotic drugs These are used to treat schizophrenia and manic episodes of bipolar depression. Older anti-psychotics cause more side effects and have been replaced by newer ones that cause fewer side effects.

Electroconvulsive (ECT) therapy

ECT is used in when depression is severe or life-threatening, or where other treatment has not worked or for persons who cannot take antidepressant medication (Strock 2000). An estimated 10,000 people undergo ECT treatment annually in the UK.

Psychological therapies (psychotherapy)

There are a number of talking therapies that can be used to assist with the treatment of depression. The most common is probably **CBT** (cognitive behavioural), which focuses on retraining negative thinking patterns that contribute to low moods. **Humanistic** or person-centred approaches focus on listening and building an empathic, non-judgemental, congruent relationship where the individual can discuss her or his problems. **Psychodynamic** treatments tend to work at deeper levels to resolve inner conflicts and are usually only introduced when the depression has significantly improved. There are also a whole range of self-help books and strategies to assist with personal management of depression, some of which are listed in the *Complete Guide to Exercising Away Stress* (Lawrence 2005).

Alternative/complementary therapies

There is a wide range of complementary therapies that can be used to assist with treatment of depression. These include: nutrition (reducing stimulants, such as coffee and alcohol); herbal medicine, such as St John's Wort (Strock (2000) cites some ongoing research); and specific meditation and relaxation techniques to alleviate stress and anxiety. At this time, there is comparatively limited research evidence to support the use of these treatments.

Exercise recommendations

There is increasing research and evidence to recommend the use of exercise and activity in the treatment of mild to moderate depression (Biddle et al. 2000; Halliwell 2005). The National Institute for Clinical Excellence (NICE) recently made the recommendation that persons with depression (mild to moderate) 'should be advised of the benefits of following a structured and supervised exercise programme of typically up to three sessions per week of moderate duration (45 minutes to one hour) for between 10 and 12 weeks' (Halliwell 2005).

However, the specific type of exercise recommended is dependent on a number of factors. Exercise professionals working with this population should conduct a detailed screening assessment and work with other healthcare professionals to identify ways of supporting the person. The severity of the condition is a primary consideration as some clients with depression are totally demotivated and even regular daily activities, such as housework, are too much. In these instances, it may well be worth their seeking counselling support to discuss and learn to manage the thoughts and feelings that may contribute to this state prior to embarking on an exercise programme. Other considerations include the side effects of specific medications on exercise and also the treatments of any other coexisting medical conditions (which can be varied). It may be that depression occurs in response to another medical condition (rheumatoid arthritis, heart disease, cancer), in which case the exercise and activity plan would need to be different from if depression presented as an isolated condition. Each of these issues should be considered prior to making any exercise prescription or recommendations. As a guideline, Durstine and Moore (2003: 317) recommend following the ACSM prescription for the general population with a more conservative approach in relation

Table 7.1	Exercise guidelines, depression			
Training guidelines	*Cardiovascular*	*Muscle strength*	*Flexibility*	*Functional*
Frequency	3–5 days a week	2 days a week	5 days a week	Promote ADL
Intensity	RPE 11–14	50–70% of 1RM	To position of mild tension, not discomfort	Activity related to daily living
Time	20–30 minutes	1–2 sets 8–12 repetitions	15–30 seconds 2–4 repetitions	
Type	Large muscles: walk, swim, cycle	Whole body approach 8–10 exercises	Whole body approach	Walking Gardening Housework

Adapted from Durstine and Moore (2003: 318).

to intensity, as inactivity, high body fat and low self-esteem may be more common in this population. (See Table 7.1)

The client's age, fitness and current activity levels will also affect the exercise recommended. As a starting point, the *Active for Health* prescription (Department of Health 2004*a* and *b*) can be offered as a preliminary target guideline for building activity to a level that can assist with the maintenance of health and promote general feelings of well-being (see Chapter 1, table 1.1).

The appropriateness of specific types of activity will be dependent on the individual and the existence of other medical conditions (obesity, high blood pressure, etc.). For example, an overweight individual would be advised to perform lower impact and non-weight-bearing activities, whereas an individual with osteoporosis or osteoarthritis would need to follow specific guidelines that account for these other conditions.

Cardiovascular exercise can contribute to the feel-good factor (release of endorphins), which can motivate the individual to take on other activities.

Muscular strength and endurance activities assist with muscle tone and shape, which can contribute to increased physical self-esteem.

Flexibility and mobility exercises assist with efficiency of movement, making daily tasks easier. Stretching also assists with relaxation and can improve posture, which in turn can have an impact on increasing confidence.

Exercise implications

- Low levels of motivation will require sensitivity and patience on the part of the trainer. When people feel depressed, they are often unmotivated to do housework or any other tasks that were previously undertaken. A supportive, encouraging and empathic approach is essential.

- Energy levels may also be low and the person may feel tired a lot of the time; therefore, intensity needs to be lower with the possibility of rests within the session or an accumulative approach to activity taken.

- The positive benefits of exercise need to be reinforced and the person must be praised for small efforts, which can make a big difference to their overall health.

- Medication can have an effect on heart rate, blood pressure and energy levels and may contribute to weight gain. All of these must be accounted for prior to recommending any specific exercise programme.

- Enjoyment and fun should be incorporated into the activity and, where possible, socialisation, for example group exercise where participants can encourage and support each other.

- The inclusion of specific relaxation techniques that the client can practise at home is useful for managing anxiety.

- Specific techniques that promote positive self-talk and affirmations are also useful to assist with the development of a positive attitude that can carry over into other areas of life.

- Frequency, intensity, time and type of activity will be determined by other individual factors already discussed.

Stress-related disorders

There is no specifically agreed definition of stress and there are a number of conditions that are considered to be stress related. These include: general anxiety disorder (GAD), post-traumatic stress disorder (PTSD), panic attacks and phobias.

General anxiety This is perhaps the most common of the stress-related conditions, as most people experience some sort of stress at some point in their lives. The main focus of this chapter is related to this condition. Other stress-related conditions are introduced briefly. General anxiety/stress can be viewed as a psychological condition that will be influenced by an individual's perceived ability to balance the demands of their environment (work, relationships, health etc.) with their internal and external coping resources (positive mental attitude, physical fitness, friends, family, finances etc.). Unhealthy stress and anxiety levels occur when a person feels unable to cope, and when s/he perceives a situation as applying an abnormal pressure that taxes and exceeds their internal and external resources (Lawrence 2005).

Panic attacks These are characterised by a sudden and overwhelming sense of fear, which brings on panic and apprehension. The person may experience laboured breathing, hyperventilation, palpitations, sweating, giddiness and nausea. Learning to breathe calmly when feeling an attack coming on can reduce most of the physical symptoms and bring back a state of calm.

Post-traumatic stress disorder PTSD is brought on by exposure to a stressful experience that is considered outside the normal range of life events, for example, being the victim of or witnessing abuse, torture, accidents and/or disasters that involve death and traumatic human suffering. Persons experiencing PTSD will relive the traumatic experience through repetitive thoughts or dreams, which cause the physical, mental and emotional responses brought on by the original event to be re-experienced. Learning to relax and reframing the experience (e.g. reducing self-blame) are key methods of treatment. Medication can sometimes be used to manage symptoms and social support can provide a sense of belonging and care that will ease the pain.

Phobias Davison and Neale (2001: 128) describe a phobia as a disrupting fear and avoidance that is out of proportion to the danger posed by the feared object/situation and which is recognised by the person as groundless.

Common phobias include: heights, animals, injections, blood, flying, lifts, open or closed spaces. Treatments range from psychoanalytic therapy, which explores repressed conflicts that are assumed to underlie the fear, to behavioural treatments that involve relaxing (hypnotising) the person and then exposing them to the trigger or getting them to visualise the trigger. Medication can also be prescribed in the form of sedatives.

Prevalence

The Mental Health Foundation suggests:

- Over 12 million people visit their GP each year for mental health problems and most are diagnosed as suffering from anxiety and depression that is stress related (Daines et al. 1997).
- The number of prescriptions for anti-depressants has almost tripled in England over the last 12 years, from 9.9 million prescriptions in 1992 to 27.7 prescriptions in 2003 (Halliwell 2005).

The *Occupational Health Statistics Bulletin* (Health and Safety Executive, 2002/3) indicates that:

- Stress, anxiety and depression were the second most commonly reported illness and individuals believed their condition was caused or made worse by their current or past work.
- The prevalence of stress and related (mainly heart) conditions has increased to double the level in 1990.
- In 2001/2 stress, depression or anxiety and musculo-skeletal disorders accounted for the majority of workdays lost.

The Health and Safety Executive (2005) report cites research studies that indicate:

- Work-related stress, anxiety and depression account for 13 million reported lost working days per year.
- 254,000 people first become aware of work-related stress, anxiety or depression in the 12 months prior to reporting it.
- Over half a million individuals in Britain believed in 2003/4 that they were experiencing work-related stress that was making them ill.

Causes

There are numerous theories regarding the causes of stress, which include those listed for depression:

- biological (brain chemistry);
- genetic disposition (heredity);
- environmental and social factors (stress, relationship problems, illness, bereavement, loss of job, life transitions etc.);
- psychoanalytic (early developmental experiences);
- cognitive-behavioural (thinking patterns);
- humanistic (low self-worth);
- family systems (relationships and roles within the family).

A combination of the above and other social and environment factors can trigger an individual to experience the stress response (fight or flight).

Work: Change of job, unemployment, redundancy, promotion, retirement.

Relationships: Marriage, divorce, birth of child, arguments with partner.

Financial: Mortgage, loans.

Life events: Death of relatives, partner or friends.

Family: Moving house, holidays, trouble with relatives.

Health: Changes in health status, diagnosis of medical condition.

Signs and symptoms of stress/anxiety

There are numerous signs and symptoms of stress, which can manifest in different ways. See table 7.2.

In instances where stress is prolonged, for example, being out of work for a long time or experiencing the effects of a debilitating condition (e.g. rheumatoid arthritis), the body has to find additional ways to cope. In such times the pituitary gland and adrenal cortex system play a greater role to ensure energy is managed to meet the extra demands. The impact of longer-term stress on the body is outlined in table 7.3.

Treatment

Medication In serious instances medication can be introduced to assist with the management of anxiety and depressive symptoms (see table 7.4). The medications prescribed for depression are also used to treat specific stress-related disorders: SSRIs for panic attacks and social phobias; tricyclics for general anxiety disorders (GAD) and panic attacks; benzodiaepines for general anxiety disorders and post-traumatic stress disorder (PTSD).

Table 7.2	Signs and symptoms of stress		
Physical	*Mental*	*Emotional*	*Behavioural*
Spots	Irrational thoughts	Sadness	Eating more or less
Shoulder tension	Mental fatigue	Depression	Drinking more stimulants
Skin disorders	Poor decision making	Anger	Smoking more
Chest pain	Low self-esteem	Fear	Swearing
Increased heart rate	Low self-worth	Panic	Aggression
Nervous indigestion	Inability to listen	Irritability	Violence
Fast, shallow breathing	Procastination	Boredom	Crime
Upper back hunched	Excessive self-criticism	Loneliness	Crying
Yawning/sighing	Egocentricity	Jealousy	Increased or decreased sexual libido
Increased blood pressure	Accident-proneness	Resentment	Excessive talking
Abdominal pain	Making more mistakes	Helplessness	Foot tapping

Adapted from *The Complete Guide to Exercising Away Stress*, Lawrence (2005).

Table 7.3	Some of the longer-term effects of stress
Long-term stress	*The effects on the body*
The hormonal system	The pituitary–adrenal cortex system is more dominant in times of long-term stress. Cortisol levels are increased to supply the energy to meet these increased demands. Excessive levels of cortisol suppress the immune system, which makes us more susceptible to illness and disease.
The immune system	Suppression of the immune system can make us more susceptible to colds and flu and diseases that effect the immune system itself, such as some cancers. Long-term stress can also affect the body's healing and repair process, which may have an impact on the health of our bones (osteoporosis) and other tissues.
The sex hormones	The sex hormones increase when we experience feeling more secure. Testosterone (and the female version androstendione) levels can increase when feelings of power, control, dominance and success are experienced in a particular situation. Levels of sex hormones can play a key role in influencing our social behaviour and relationships (support systems). Suppression of the reproductive system can lead to cessation of menstruation in women, impotence in men and loss of libido in both genders.
The respiratory system	The effects of long-term stress triggers on the respiratory system may be to induce and increase the symptoms of asthma and other respiratory conditions.
The digestive system	Suppression of the digestive system may lead to diseases such as constipation, diarrhoea, irritable bowel etc.
The heart and circulatory system	Excess blood sugars may contribute to furring of the artery walls (atherosclerosis), which may lead to coronary artery disease.
Other systems:	Long-term stress can have an effect on managing blood sugar levels and may be linked to adult onset diabetes.

From: *The Complete Guide to Exercising Away Stress*, Lawrence (2005).

Self-help There are numerous self-help books available to assist with management of stress, anxiety and panic. Some self-help strategies (positive thinking, relaxation techniques, goal-setting, time management, assertiveness) are discussed in *The Complete Guide to Exercising Away Stress* (Lawrence 2005).

Breathing and relaxation There is a tendency towards shallow and rapid breathing, using mainly the upper thorax or chest (where the upper chest and shoulders lift and lower as we breathe). Poor breathing habits such as these can contribute to anxiety and panic, and are more common in people who are sedentary.

Ideally, we should use the whole of the ribcage and abdomen when we breathe (diaphragm and abdominal breathing). Focusing on deeper and slower breathing can help to reduce the immediate and long-term effects of the fight and flight response and can help return the body to a more natural unstressed state.

Breathing exercise

- Take the breath slightly deeper into the lower ribcage (most people take very shallow breaths into the upper chest area only).
- Keep the breath soft, smooth and rhythmical.
- Find a natural breathing pace.
- Find a natural breathing power (not forcing or straining).
- Let the breath become effortless and allow it to flow freely.
- Notice the abdomen rise and fall.
- Allow the breath to quiet and calm the mind.
- Allow a few minutes just to focus on the breathing and stillness.

Counselling and psychotherapy Each of the therapies listed for depression are appropriate for exploring stress. Therapists should be registered with either BACP or UKCP.

Alternative therapies Nutrition, massage, homeopathy and acupuncture can all contribute to managing stress.

Relaxation One technique for promoting relaxation is the Benson method. Herbert Benson developed it for people with high blood pressure. He initially suggested that individuals sit still and quiet and focus on saying the word 'one' on their outward breath for a short duration of time, just letting the mind and body slow down with no specific effort.

The technique can be adapted in the following ways:

- The word 'one' can be replaced by other words that an individual may find more natural, such as: calm, peace, love, still, silent, relax, etc.
- The word can be spoken silently within, rather than out loud.
- The technique can be used in everyday activities, for example: when queuing at a supermarket, on the train, while out walking, at an office desk, etc.

Adapted version of Benson method relaxation script

Sit quietly with an open body posture.
Focus on the breathing.
As you breathe out, focus on a desired word (calm, one, peace, relax, joy).
The word can be spoken out loud or quietly within.
Practice this for about five minutes, just allowing the body to relax.

Exercise recommendations

Stress may be the most common of the mental health conditions; it is certainly the one that most people would report experiencing. With this in mind, it is advised that ACSM guidelines for the general population (Chapter 2) are used to prescribe a programme of exercise and activity. However, specific training recommendations for frequency, intensity, time and type (FITT) should be prescribed and considered in relation to each of the following:

- the existing fitness level and activity levels of the individual;
- the severity and length of experiencing of their stress-related condition;
- personal circumstances and support systems;
- previous and current medical history;
- existence of other medical conditions that may be medicated;
- medications.

Table 7.4	Some example medications and their impact on exercise

Antidepressants		
Drug category and name	*Side effects*	*Exercise implications*
Selective serotonin uptake inhibitors Fluoxetine (Prozac) Fluvoxamine (Faverin) Sertraline (Lustrol) Paroxetine (Seroxat) Citalopram (Cipramil)	Nausea Vomiting Insomnia Drowsiness Anxiety, restlessness Sexual dysfunction Fatigue Headaches Gastrointestinal complaints	Poor coordination Drowsiness Fatigue Increased heart rate Tremors Impaired memory Work at lower intensity Use RPE
Tricyclics Amitriptyline Clomipramine Dosulepin (Dothiepin) Imipramine Lofepramine	Drowsiness Constipation Dry mouth Blurred vision Weight gain Hypotension Erectile failure Heart attack Stroke	Balance problems Poor body image Dizziness Slowed reactions
Monoamine oxidase inhibitors (MAOIs) Isocarboxazid Moclobemide Phenelzine	Increased blood pressure Headache and vomiting when taken with tyramine-rich foods Dizziness Dry mouth	Increased blood pressure Increased heart rate Use RPE Work at lower intensity
Anxiolytics (Sedatives)		
Benzodiazepines Diazepam (Valium) Chlordiazepoxide (Librium) Temazepam	Drowsiness Dizziness Ataxia Headache	Poor concentration Postural hypotension Balance abnormalities Slowed reactions

Table 7.4	Some example medications and their impact on exercise cont.	
	Anxiolytics (Sedatives)	
Drug category and name	Side effects	Exercise implications
Benzodiazepines cont. Oxazepam Lorazepam (Ativan) Nitrazepam (Mogodon)	Blurred vision Forgetfulness Confusion	Lethargy Dizziness Reduced heart rate Reduced respiration rate Use RPE Work at lower intensity Avoid quick movement changes
Beta-blockers Propranolol Atenolol Oxprenolol	Cold extremities Aching muscles Fatigue Fainting	Fatigue Aching muscles Reduced heart rate Reduced blood pressure Use RPE scale Will need increased duration but decreased intensity

MUSCULAR AND SKELETAL CONDITIONS

8

Muscular and skeletal conditions are those that affect the muscular system and/or skeletal system and contribute to a reduction in mobility, bringing about physical limitations. The conditions discussed in this chapter are:

- Osteoporosis
- Osteoarthritis
- Total hip replacement
- Rheumatoid arthritis
- Low back pain.

Osteoporosis

Osteoporosis is often referred to as brittle bone disease. It occurs when the bones suffer a loss in calcium and other mineral content, which contributes to their becoming more porous and as a consequence more brittle. This makes the bones more susceptible to breaking when put under the stress of what may constitute a normal living activity for a person with a healthy bone mass.

The World Health Organisation (WHO) differentiates between osteopenia and osteoporosis by defining them as follows:

- Osteopenia: Bone mineral density >1 standard deviation below young normal values
- Osteoporosis: Bone mineral density >2.5 standard deviation below young normal values (Bloomfield and Smith 1991).

These definitions are used in clinical diagnosis.

Prevalence

The density of bones builds to a peak level until the age of 30, after which bone mass begins to deteriorate at a rate of approximately 1 per cent per year (depending on other lifestyle factors, as listed below).

A loss of bone density (osteopenia) is therefore evident from a comparatively young age. Women develop bone loss more quickly than men: approximately three times faster. This rate increases during the menopause, when there is an evident reduction of the hormone oestrogen, which influences bone mass. The National Osteoporosis Society (2005) reports that by the time some women reach the age of 70 they have lost anything up to 30 per cent of their bone. They also suggest that one in three women and one in 12 men over 50 will fracture a bone due to osteoporosis. The Chief Medical Office report, 'At Least Five a Week' (2005: 54), suggests that there are 'around 60,000 osteoporotic hip fractures in the UK each year' and that '15–20 per cent of those people with fractures will die within a year from causes related to the fracture'.

Causes

Loss of bone density, or mineral mass, is to some extent a process that is related to the unchangeable factor of ageing. However, there are numerous other genetic and lifestyle factors, some of which are changeable, others that are not, which contribute to the maintenance of a comparatively healthy bone density (McArdle, Katch and Katch 1991: 54; Bloomfield and Smith 2003: 222). These include:

- Gender: females are more susceptible than men due to hormonal changes.
- Age: loss of bone density increases with seniority; men are less susceptible to clinically significant changes before the age of 70, but other lifestyle factors impact this.
- Hormones: women who experience an early menopause (before age 45) are more susceptible due to a reduction in the hormone oestrogen. Men with low testosterone levels are more at risk. The worst combination for bone health is late onset of menstruation combined with early menopause (CMO 2005: 54).
- Heredity: women with a maternal parent experiencing the condition are more susceptible.
- Diet: diets lacking sufficient intake of calcium and vitamin D; diets with excessive intake of caffeine, alcohol, and carbonated drinks increase risk as these reduce calcium absorption.
- Body type: slender body frames are more susceptible.
- Sedentary lifestyle: inactivity or lack of weight-bearing exercise contributes to the rate at which the skeleton ages. Muscles pull on bones; this increases blood flow and the delivery of nutrients (calcium). Inactivity and lack of use of specific muscles will affect the density of the specific bones in the less-used areas. Persons with lower muscle mass and lower muscle strength are at risk of lower bone density.
- Smoking: smoking effects the calcification and consequently the mineral content of bones.
- Anorexia and prolonged amenorrhoea (pre- and post-menopause): interruptions to monthly cycles (periods) affect hormone levels and bone density.
- Ethnicity: Caucasian and Asian women are more susceptible.
- Medication: some medications contribute to losses of bone density (corticosteroids and anticonvulsants)
- Nulliparity: Women who have never experienced a pregnancy are also more at risk, since hormone levels rise during pregnancy.

Signs and symptoms

Osteoporosis can develop steadily and progressively over several years without any observable signs or symptoms. Osteopenia and osteoporosis are both becoming more prevalent, therefore some conscious awareness-raising of the risk factors (via education) associated with the condition is essential for persons to identify their potential risk(s) and make appropriate lifestyle changes to prevent deterioration becoming more rapid.

In most instances the first indication of osteoporosis is a fracture to a bone that occurs as a result of a falling accident, which would not occur in a younger person experiencing the same fall or accident. Typical areas of breakage are the wrist and hip joints and the spine.

In more severe cases of osteoporosis, there may be evidence of changes to the spinal curvatures, in particular of the thoracic spine. As the vertebrae lose density they crumble, which leads progressively to a decrease in height and contributes to an increased kyphotic curve of the thoracic spine, giving a hunchback appearance (kyphosis). This occurs because of an increased anterior pressure on the vertebrae, which contributes to a wedge-shaped crushing. Kyphosis reduces the mobility in that area of the spine and may also contribute to breathing problems, as the ribs attach with the thoracic spine, and it is the contraction of the intercostal muscles (attached to the ribs) and the diaphragm muscle (lying underneath the ribcage like a hammock) that assists breathing. These factors may also contribute to fractures occurring to the ribs and vertebrae in response to coughing (in severe cases). An extreme kyphotic posture can also increase the risk of falls, because the rounding forward of the spine creates a change in the centre of gravity, which affects the person's balance, stability and coordination.

Treatment

Treatment and management of the condition will be dependent on its severity. Brewer et al. (2003: 97) cite three categories of osteoporotic patients:

- **Group one** Persons with normal bone mass with other lifestyle factors that may contribute to reduction in bone mass, and persons with mild changes in bone density (osteopenia).
- **Group two** Persons with a clinical diagnosis of osteoporosis without a history of fracture.
- **Group three** Persons with advanced changes in bone density with a history of fracture, most commonly the frail and elderly population.

For the first group, the aim of any treatment programme should be to reduce the lifestyle risk factors associated with loss of bone density and to maintain and where possible increase the density of the bone and prevent premature deterioration.

For the second group, the aim of a treatment programme is similar to that of the first group. However, there may be evidence of medical interventions such as hormone replacement therapy for post-menopausal women and any

exercise prescription should be offered with greater sensitivity to individual needs, the progressive state of the condition and the increased risk of fractures and falls.

For the third group, the primary aim is to reduce the risk of falls and maintain levels of mobility and bone and muscle strength. Exercise prescription for this group would need to be more considerate of postural and balance changes, lack of mobility and strength and the comparatively low fitness level and tolerance to exercise apparent in this group.

Hormone replacement therapy and the use of specific drugs such as bisphosphonates can be part of the treatment plan. However, they are not usually recommended as the first line of treatment for women over 50. They may be recommended when other treatments are ineffective, cannot be tolerated or are contraindicated. Calcitonin may be considered for those at high risk of osteoporosis and for whom bisphosphonates are unsuitable.

Other recommendations would be to reduce and manage specific lifestyle behaviour factors (e.g. reduce smoking, manage activities, etc.).

Exercise recommendations and limitations

For all groups, the progressive stage of the condition will influence the specific recommendations for exercise and activity. For example: a person with mild changes in bone density with fewer contributory risk factors (e.g. smoking) may require a different exercise programme from a person with similar changes of bone density but more contributory risk factors (e.g. smoking, sedentary lifestyle, poor heredity, post-menopausal). The aim of exercise as an intervention at this stage of the condition would be more as a preventative measure to reduce the risk of the condition deteriorating too rapidly. As a general rule, persons from this preventative group would be able to perform exercises and activities that are comparatively more challenging than would a person where the condition is more progressive, for example a person recently clinically diagnosed with osteoporosis after experiencing a fracture or a frailer, elderly person.

Some general aims for working with these populations

1. Provide education and support that will promote a reduction in the lifestyle factors that contribute to the condition, and;

2. Reduce the risk of falls, in the present or in the future, by focusing on training the following physical components:

- **Muscular strength training** The aim of this should be to improve the overall strength of the muscles, with a focus on site-specific training and weight-bearing activities for areas more vulnerable to fractures, such as wrist, hip, spine and collarbone. Body-weight exercises such as press-ups or squats, or resistance machines such as chest press and leg press, will add to the load borne by these areas. A combination of strength work for the lower body and balance work is most successful at decreasing the risk of falls. Therefore, it is wise to include specific exercises to improve posture and balance and maintain the strength of the vertebral bones. Pilates-based exercise focuses on working the core muscles and can be beneficial. Other exercises to strengthen the muscles of the abdominals and back extensors are also appropriate. Strengthening of the back extensors is particularly important, so they can act as a splint to the crumbling spine. Any specific strength exercises recommended should be relative to the ability and starting level of the individual.

- **Mobility and flexibility** The focus of mobility and flexibility work should be to maintain or improve the condition of those muscles that contribute to changes in posture. Stretching of the pectoral muscles can help to improve or prevent kyphotic posture.

- **Cardiovascular training** Any specific recommendations for cardiovascular exercise and/or activity should take into account the individual's ability and current level of exercise and fitness. The aim should be to maintain existing fitness and, where possible, make improvements.

Any specific exercise recommendation would need to take the following into account:

- the existing fitness level and activity levels of the individual;

- the severity and longevity of experiencing the condition (this may have an impact on psychological well-being and contribute to depression or anxiety);

- personal circumstances and support systems;

- previous and current medical history;

- existence of other medical conditions that may be medicated and may present further considerations regarding exercise type and intensity;

- the exercise setting (the programme may be offered in a gym or in a residential home for the elderly);

- individual factors: age, gender, lifestyle and other associated risk factors.

For the at-risk group (group one) Traditional weight-bearing activity and exercise are appropriate, although age, current fitness and activity levels and exercise experience also need to be taken into account. Some higher-impact work may be appropriate for this group, such as jogging, skipping and aerobic dancing to improve cardiovascular fitness and strengthen the lower body. Again, the type of activity recommended will be dependent on the factors previously mentioned. Strength training for specific body areas can also be included, for example: back extensions and other postural and abdominal core stability exercises (such as those performed in pilates) to strengthen the muscles around the spine.

- Chest presses, chest flyes, press-ups or other exercises bearing the weight of the upper body (such as reciprocal reach of arms – a Pilates exercise) strengthen the chest and arms and create bone loading of the wrists and collarbones.

- Lateral leg raises strengthen the muscles and load the bones around the hip and pelvis. Hopping and jumping movements will also contribute to strengthening these muscles, but are higher impact in nature and should be used only if appropriate for the individual.

- Leg presses, squatting and walking will strengthen the muscles and load the bones of the lower body and are appropriate.

- Reverse flyes and some Pilates-based exercises strengthen the muscles and load the bones around the shoulder girdle, which can also contribute to improvements in any apparent kyphosis.

For the clinically diagnosed group (group two) More care and attention may need to be provided regarding the specific exercises recommended. The focus towards training those areas of the body suggested above still apply, except the workload might have to be comparatively lower. Any cardiovascular exercise may need to be lower impact, such as walking and some aerobic dance classes involving marches, grapevines, etc. Some attention should also be given regarding the appropriateness of specific exercise positions.

For the frailer groups (group three) This group will most likely have a lower tolerance for exercise and activity. The likelihood of falling and consequent apprehensiveness may be also be apparent. These factors, in addition to others mentioned for the previous groups (age, other medical conditions, etc.) will dramatically affect the type and intensity of any exercise and activity recommended. One of the primary aims for working with this group is to reduce the risk of falls by developing motor skills and strength of related muscles.

Stretching and strengthening exercises Exercises to assist with posture and improve the mobility of the thoracic spine and the mobility and flexibility of the upper body are appropriate (trunk rotations, side bends, shoulder girdle retractions, abdominal hollowing). However, the range of motion may need to be reduced and the speed of movement slowed down; in some instances there may be no or very little range of movement (e.g. spine rotation) and so care must be taken, especially if the person presents with kyphosis that is due to bone deterioration. Weight-bearing positions where the body is lying on the floor are probably totally inappropriate, particularly if the condition is advanced. Alternative exercises that enable these movements can be performed from a seated position, for example: seated back extensions and spine rotations, or simply sitting upright in a chair. Gentle lateral breathing exercises (as used in Pilates) can also help to improve mobility of the thoracic area.

Chair-based sessions The focus in these sessions is on improving mobility, flexibility and strength and the opportunity to take a rest is easily available. These sessions can include activities that relate to daily functions, such as getting up and down from a seated position, reaching down to the side to lift something from the floor while seated, and wrist-strengthening exercises with exercise bands to assist with unscrewing jars or buttoning shirts/blouses. A further benefit of these exercises is that they also target key potential fracture sites.

Exercise in water Some very gentle mobility exercises and strengthening exercises in water can be beneficial. However, the water should be warm to prevent chilling and the exercise performed at chest depth to maximise buoyancy and promote flotation, which contribute to relieving weight-bearing and can assist with easing and improving range of motion. The main disadvantage, however, is that the non-weight-bearing nature of this exercise is less effective at loading bones. Even so, the muscles still have to pull on bones and this will still have some strengthening effect. Another consideration would be that the hydrostatic pressure of the water could press against the ribcage and make breathing more conscious. This may create an additional risk for persons with breathing and respiratory problems (e.g. asthma, COPD).

Cardiovascular training Any cardiovascular activity will need to be of a considerably lower intensity with this group, especially since, for some, a simple cough may cause a rib to break. For those capable and able, a very gentle walking programme or some very gentle exercise in water may be appropriate.

Exercise implications

- Avoid forward flexion performed alone or combined with twisting movements as this may contribute to vertebral fractures.
- Avoid high-impact work with clinically diagnosed osteoporotic subjects.
- Prone and supine lying positions may be inappropriate for persons susceptible to vertebral fractures; use standing and seated alternatives.

Table 8.1	Exercise guidelines, osteoporosis			
Training guidelines	Cardiovascular	Muscle strength	Flexibility	Functional
Frequency	3–5 days a week	2–3 days a week	5–7 days a week	2–5 days a week
Intensity	40–70% of HRmax	75% of 1RM	To position of mild tension discomfort.	Activity related to daily living.
Time	20–30 minutes	2 sets 8–10 reps	Develop or maintain range of motion.	
Type	Large muscles. Walk, swim, cycle	Upper body (arms and shoulders). Lower body (legs). Trunk (abdominals and back extensors).	Focus on pectorals and other muscles that affect posture.	Walking. Sit to stand. Lifting correctly without spine flexion. Balance.

Adapted from Durstine and Moore (2003: 226).

- Persons with extreme kyphosis may be able to walk only with support (to prevent falls) so alternative modes of cardiovascular training, such as a recumbent cycle, may be more appropriate, as this offers some support to the body.

- Ensure environment is free of obstacles to reduce anxiety about falling.

- If weight-bearing exercise is not possible, select chair-based or water-based exercise programmes.

- Target fracture sites (hip, wrist, collarbone).

- Certain medications may cause uncomfortable side effects and these should be considered prior to making specific exercise recommendations to the individual.

- Any further doubts or concerns should always be discussed with the client's physiotherapist.

- Be aware of other medical conditions (CHD etc.) in more sedentary and senior clients.

See also table 8.1.

Osteoarthritis

Osteoarthritis is a degenerative condition of the joints that is most commonly brought on by the natural wear and tear associated with daily living and moving.

The articular cartilage in the affected joints becomes roughened and eventually thinner (worn down), which makes joint movement less easy and sometimes painful. As the condition worsens, the body attempts to compensate for this thinning: first, the outer edges of the bones thicken and change shape, and bony outgrowths called osteophytes form at the outer edges. Then the membranes lining the joint can become inflamed. This makes movement more uncomfortable, increases pain further and can lead to inflammation and swelling around the joint. In severe cases, calcium can be laid down in the cartilage (calcification), hardening it further.

The primary joints affected are the weight-bearing joints of the body, which include:

- knees
- hips
- lumbar area of the spine
- wrists and hands.

Prevalence

The National Institute of Arthritis and Musculoskeletal and Skin Diseases (2002) suggests that osteoarthritis is more common in men before the age of 45 and more common in women after the age of 45. This may be influenced by a higher participation in sporting activities by men or maybe the types of activities they take part in (rugby, football and boxing), which, while not exclusive to men, do tend to be male-dominated. NIAMS (2002) also suggests that over 20 million people in the USA have the disease and suggests it is a frequent cause of disability among the adult population.

Causes

The causes of arthritis are not yet known (NIAMS 2002). However, it is believed that the following are all contributory factors:

- Ageing brings the culmination of natural wear and tear and is a primary cause and risk, although there are cases of osteoarthritis in younger age groups.

- Being heavily overweight or obese increases the stress on the joints and can contribute to deterioration.

- Injury to the joints makes highly active sportspeople more susceptible.

- Overuse of the joints, including excessive and repetitive joint movements or positions (such as excessive kneeling), may make it more prevalent in specific types of occupation.
- A family history of osteoarthritis increases the risk.

Signs and symptoms

A combination of examinations would need to be performed for clinical diagnosis and may include: physical examination, clinical history, x-ray, etc.

The signs and symptoms of osteoarthritis can sometimes include:

- steady or intermittent pain in the affected joints;
- discomfort or stiffness when moving the joint(s);
- reduction and limitation to range of motion;
- inflammation and tenderness;
- a crunching or creaking feeling when moving the joint(s);
- joint instability and weakness in surrounding muscles;
- joint deformity.

The impact of the condition on lifestyle and limitations to mobility can also contribute to feelings of helplessness, anxiety and depression.

Treatment

Prevention or reduction of the factors that may contribute to arthritis is the first line of treatment: maintaining an ideal body-weight; being active to maintain a wide range of motion in joints and maintain strength of surrounding muscles to assist joint stability; avoiding extremes of activity where the joint(s) may be overstressed, such as prolonged kneeling or excessive impact, or some sports; wearing shock-absorbing insoles in shoes or trainers, are all ways of preventing deterioration. In severe cases, using a walking aid assists with weight-bearing.

Medication

There is a range of medications used to treat osteoarthritis. These aim to reduce pain and limit deterioration in the joints, maintaining their functionality. GPs may prescribe in the first instance a pain reliever such as paracetamol and in some cases stronger pain killers such as co-codamol or co-dydramol, which are a combination of paracetamol and codeine.

If the joint becomes inflamed, non-steroidal anti-inflammatory drugs may be prescribed (NSAID), such as ibuprofen. These medications have anti-inflammatory and analgesic properties to reduce pain, swelling and stiffness in the joints. However, these can sometimes cause side effects, which include indigestion, diarrhoea and gastro-intestinal bleeding. These medications could also trigger an asthma attack in asthmatics.

In more extreme cases where the joint(s) become very painful, localised corticosteroid injections can be effective for reducing pain and swelling. However, Minor and Kay (2003) suggest that these injections should not be administered too frequently as they can cause tissue destruction. The type and intensity of activity after an injection would also need to be considered. In some instances, no exercise should occur for two weeks following an injection.

Surgery

In extreme cases, surgery can be used as a treatment. Hip replacements are usually effective for about ten years and can bring about improved mobility and pain reduction.

Knee replacements are more complex, but again can eventually improve mobility and reduce pain.

As with all surgery, there are risks associated that are similar for most major surgical procedures.

Exercise

Although certain types of exercise may be contraindicated, it is generally recommended to keep the joints moving. Mobility and flexibility exercises will help to maintain and improve range of motion. Muscular strength and endurance activities will help to strengthen the muscles around the joints, to maintain or improve joint stability. These exercises can also assist with reducing pain. Cardiovascular activities are important to maintain fitness of the heart and lungs and prevent coronary heart disease etc., which can lead to further disability. The type of activity selected will be dependent on the severity of the condition and other factors specific to the individual, for example: age, previous exercise and activity levels, other medical conditions and medications etc. A general recommendation would be for cardiovascular activities to be non-weight-bearing for the specific affected joint(s).

Exercise recommendations and limitations

Some general guidelines for working with persons with osteoarthritis include:

- **Mobility and flexibility** exercises will maintain joint mobility and range of motion. The range of motion, speed and repetitions for each movement will need to be adapted for the specific individual, to accommodate the severity of the condition. These exercises can be performed in a weight-bearing position if comfortable, or can be performed on a chair to reduce weight-bearing. They can also be performed in a non-weight-bearing environment, such as a swimming pool. Exercising in chest-depth water offers the body buoyancy, supporting its weight and making movement of the joints much easier and more comfortable, thereby allowing joint movement to be increased while in the water. Exercise in water can also help to reduce swelling around the joint (Lawrence 2004a).

- **Strengthening exercises** It is essential to condition the muscles sufficiently in order to maintain joint stability. Muscle conditioning work is also essential before increasing the workload of any other activities, although again this will be dependent on the individual and factors specific to him or her (current fitness and activity levels etc.). Weight-bearing exercises do not have to be excluded, but consideration must be given to the severity of the condition. For example, the performance of squatting movements (as in sit to stand) may be comfortable for some people if the speed of the movement is controlled, repetitions limited, and the individual works to a range of motion that is comfortable for them with correct alignment. A benefit of this type of exercise is that it is functional and relates to activities the person would need for daily living. However, this type of exercise may be totally inappropriate for a person with more progressive arthritis in the knee joint, and an alternative strengthening exercise such as leg extensions (using fixed-resistance machines or bands or trainer resistance) may be more appropriate. Additionally, it may be worth starting with isometric exercises (no or small range of movement) and progressing to isotonic exercises (full range of movement), increasing the repetitions gradually (one repetition at a time) and monitoring any increase in pain occurring after exercise (> 2 hours). If weight-bearing activities are too uncomfortable, chair-based strengthening exercises can be an alternative; so too can specific water-based strength exercises.

All exercise and activities used should be low impact in nature as high-impact work increases stress on the joints. In addition, the repetitions of specific joint movements need to be reduced to avoid overuse and repetitive strain. The speed of exercise and range of motion should always be adapted to suit the individual's ability.

- **Cardiovascular activities** It is important to maintain cardiovascular fitness (health of the heart and lungs) and prevent associated conditions (high blood pressure, CHD etc.). The exercises and activities should be low impact, such as walking, cycling, swimming or exercise in water. However, care must be taken to avoid over-repetition. Thus, it may be advisable for some to accumulate activity over the day and follow the activity for health guidelines suggested in Chapter 1, table 1.1.

Table 8.2	Exercise guidelines, osteoarthritis			
Training guidelines	Cardiovascular	Muscle strength	Flexibility	Functional
Frequency	3–5 days a week	2–3 days a week	1–2 sessions a day	As is comfortable to improve quality of life.
Intensity	60–80% of HRmax RPE 11–16 on Borg (6–20 scale). This will be dependent on individual factors and any other medical conditions.	Work to individual's pain tolerance. Low resistance.	To position of mild tension, not discomfort. Pain-free range of motion.	Activity related to daily living.
Time	5 min building to 30 min. Progress duration more than intensity. Activity can be accumulated if necessary.	2–3 reps building to 10–12 reps. Dependent on above.	Avoid overstretching and avoid over-repetition of some mobility work. Aim for comfort.	
Type	Large muscles. Walk, swim, cycle. Low impact only. Vary activities to avoid repetitive strain and overuse.	Resistance machines. Circuit weight-training exercises (as appropriate). Isometric strength work on affected joints. Exercise bands or trainer-assisted resistance activities.	Stretching and regular mobility exercises. Can be chair-based, controlled range of movement.	Walking. Sit to stand. Chair-based mobility exercises.

Adapted from Durstine and Moore (2003: 212).

Exercise implications

- High-impact activities and contact sports should be avoided.
- Use correct footwear and shock-absorbing insoles for any weight-bearing activities.
- Excessive repetitions of same joint movement, particularly weight-bearing (step machines, high repetition resistance training) should also be avoided. In some instances, excessive cycling can aggravate the condition, and cross-training methods are more effective to vary joint stress.
- Prolonged activities in the same exercise position, such as kneeling or resting on all fours, should be avoided. If these activities are included, regular rests should be offered. Alternatively, a hand weight with a flattened edge can be held to support the all-fours position to maintain wrist alignment, as opposed to resting on the palms of the hands.
- Avoid activities where direction changes are excessive or fast.
- Reduce intensity and duration of exercise and/or use a different activity mode (e.g. exercise in water) if joint pain or swelling appears or continues.
- Side effects of any medications should be considered prior to making specific exercise recommendations to the individual.
- Other medical conditions, such as depression or CHD in cases of prolonged inactivity, would also need to be considered.

Any further doubts or concerns should always be discussed with the client's GP. See also table 8.2.

Total hip replacement

A hip replacement or other joint replacement is a surgical procedure used to replace a joint (partially or fully) where disease (e.g. osteoarthritis) has worn down the joint tissue. Total hip replacement can be effective in relieving pain and improving function of the joint for approximately ten years (Prodigy 2005*d*).

A new joint will be unstable and more susceptible to dislocation for a few weeks after the operation, thus great care must be taken when moving. During the post-operative phase, patients will be guided by a health professional regarding the type of activity and movement needed to assist their rehabilitation. Most people are back to normal functioning within six months, provided that no other complications present.

Exercise recommendations

- Walking;
- gentle cycling;
- low range of motion in all hip movements;
- low resistance;
- progress steadily;
- strengthen muscles around hip joint: hip flexors, hip extensors (gluteus maximus), adductors and abductors;
- exercise in water (deep water).

Exercise limitations

- For hip replacement, only limited abduction will be possible.
- Avoid adduction across the midline of the body.
- Hip flexion should be encouraged only to hip height (not more than 90 degrees).
- Avoid breaststroke leg action when swimming.
- Seated exercises can be performed in a chair where the buttocks are positioned slightly higher than the knees (a more comfortable joint angle at the hip).

- Static contractions to strengthen abductors can be appropriate (seated outer thigh exercise using resistance band or hands to resist movement).

Rheumatoid arthritis

Rheumatoid arthritis is an auto-immune disease that causes chronic inflammation. Auto-immune diseases occur when the antibodies produced by the body's immune system, which normally fight foreign substances such as viruses and bacteria, attack other tissues in the body because they identify them as foreign tissue. Rheumatoid arthritis is also referred to as a systemic disease because it affects multiple organs in the body, not just the joints.

The joints most affected are the smaller joints of the wrists, hands, fingers and toes, although as a systemic condition, it can occur anywhere in the body. In some instances the chronic inflammation can destroy other joint tissues such as cartilage, bone, ligaments and tendons, which causes the joints to become swollen, painful, stiff and sometimes deformed.

Prevalence

The disease is three times more common in women than men and can begin at any age, although it most commonly occurs between the ages of forty and sixty. It affects approximately 2–3 per cent of the adult population (Brewer et al. 2003).

Cause

The causes of rheumatoid arthritis are unknown; however, it is suspected that certain infections or triggers in the environment may cause the body to attack its own tissues (Sheil n.d.).

Signs and symptoms

When the body tissues are inflamed (flare up) the condition is considered to be active and when inflammation subsides the condition is considered to be in remission. During a flare-up the symptoms can include:

- fatigue
- loss of appetite
- muscle aches
- fever
- joint stiffness after periods of inactivity (particularly in the morning)
- red, swollen and painful joints, which in severe cases can become deformed.

Rheumatoid arthritis is a systemic disease and is not isolated to the joints. It can cause inflammation of other tissues around the eyes and other vital organs of the body such as the heart, lungs, etc.

It is essential to be aware of emotional and mental symptoms in addition to the physical symptoms. The disability and deformity that can be caused by the condition can impact daily activities (work etc.) quite significantly and can contribute to feelings of emotional distress, hopelessness, anxiety and depression.

Treatment

The main goal of any treatment is to:

- reduce joint inflammation and pain;
- prevent destruction and deformity of the joints;
- maintain joint functionality.

Treatment usually involves a combination of medication, joint strengthening exercises and mobility and rest. In severe cases surgery can be used to restore joint mobility, repair damage to joints and sometimes replace joints with artificial materials. The use of support groups and counselling can also help individuals to manage the emotional stress, discuss problems associated with changes to their physical condition and provide education about their illness.

Medication

Aspirin and ibuprofen (NSAIDS) are the fast-acting first line of treatment, as are corticosteroids, which reduce swelling and pain. The side effects of corticosteroids include thinning of the skin and bone (which adds the risk of osteoporosis), weight gain (which can place further stress on the joints, if unmanaged) and easier bruising. Disease-modifying anti-rheumatic drugs (DMARDS) are the slower-acting second line of drug treatment, which aims to prevent the progressive destruction to the joint tissues and, if effective, promote the remission phase of the condition.

Exercise

Regular exercise plays an important role in maintaining joint mobility and strength of the muscles around the joint. However, the degree of joint destruction will affect the type of exercise that can be performed. Painful joints should be rested and not exercised during a flare-up, but once pain eases, stretching and mobility exercises, gentle weight-training to increase muscle strength and cardiovascular activities such as swimming and cycling can be performed. Exercise in water is particularly beneficial as water offers support to the body and the increased buoyancy minimises stress on the joints. Water also adds a resistance to movement that can be utilised to increase muscular strength and cardiovascular gains. Managing body-weight and losing excess weight can prevent additional stress on the joints.

Exercise recommendations

The most essential point is that *no* exercise should be performed on the affected joints when the condition is active (in a flare-up phase) because this may worsen the damage. During a remission phase, exercise and activity can resume with a focus on maintaining joint mobility and range of motion and maintaining or increasing strength of the muscles around the joint. However, the speed of movement, range of motion, repetitions and any resistance must be adapted to suit the individual's ability. In most cases, the intensity (repetitions, rate, ROM, resistance) of any exercise will need to start low and progress gradually.

The exercise guidelines offered for osteo-arthritis can be applied to rheumatoid arthritis. Again, particular consideration needs to be given to the severity of the condition and limitation of movement in damaged or deformed joints before recommending any specific exercise or activity.

Exercise limitations

- Never exercise the affected joints during a flare-up as this may cause further damage to the joint structure.

- Be considerate to any past damage to the joints as this may affect the intensity, range of motion and speed of movement that is achievable.

- During remission periods work on maintaining strength of muscles around the joint and working through full range of motion.

- Avoid high-impact activities or contact sports.

- Avoid excessive repetitions of same joint movement.

- Some exercise positions may not be appropriate, for example resting on all fours will be uncomfortable for wrists.

- Avoid fast-paced movements and/or quick changes of direction.

- Advise exercise in the afternoon or evening to avoid morning stiffness.

- Reduce intensity and duration of exercise and/or use a different activity mode (e.g. exercise in water) if joint pain or swelling appears or continues.

- Side effects of any medications should be considered prior to making specific exercise recommendations to the individual.

- Emotional and stress-related conditions, such as depression, that may occur in response to the condition should be considered.

- The risk of CHD in cases of prolonged inactivity should be considered.

- An occupational therapist or physiotherapist may use splint supports to assist performance of some movements. Sometimes devices to assist with lifestyle activities, such as jar grippers and toilet-seat lifters, are used to assist with daily activities.

Any further doubts or concerns should always be discussed with the client's GP.

Simple low back pain

Prodigy (2005c) defines simple low back pain as that 'in which the cause of the pain cannot be attributed to any other specific pathology'.

Low back pain is very common and most people experience some kind of simple low back pain at some point in their lives. Although most is not due to any serious disease, low back pain can contribute to a restriction in movement that makes daily activities less comfortable and sometimes more difficult. The pain can vary from severe, long-term, to mild, short-lived. Low back pain will usually resolve within a few weeks for most people; however, episodes can be recurrent.

The lower back is made up of five bones (the lumbar vertebrae). Between these bones are the inter-vertebral discs that act as shock absorbers and allow for motion of the lumbar spine. Behind the discs runs the spinal canal, which carries the spinal nerves. At the back of the spine are the spinous processes. These are the attachment points for all the muscles surrounding the spine, which move and stabilise the spine.

Prevalence

The CMO (2005: 56) report, 'At Least Five a Week', claims that 80 per cent of people in the UK experience low back pain at some point in their lives, with an estimated 150 million working days being lost each year due to low back pain. It occurs equally between men and women and most commonly between the ages of 30 and 50 and accounts for approximately 4 per cent of visits to the GP (Prodigy 2005c).

Causes

The exact causes of low back pain are not clearly understood; however, a number of lifestyle factors may contribute to the risk. The Health and Safety Executive (Prodigy 2005c) lists the following as the most-reported risk factors contributing to low back pain:

- manual handling (lifting and carrying of heavy loads, which includes lifting people and also resistances that are positioned awkwardly);

- awkward postures and movements, which include bending, twisting and static postures; poor positioning of desks, chairs and work stations which contribute to postural mis-alignment;

- whole body vibration (which can occur when truck driving or drilling);

- heavy physical work (building and labouring);
- heavy sporting activities (weight-lifting) can have an adverse effect on the spine while reducing low back pain.

Other factors may include ageing, general ill health, height (and maybe weight, which can affect posture). Pregnancy may contribute to back pain (due to postural misalignment), as can psychological factors (lack of self-esteem, self-worth, satisfaction, confidence etc., all of which can influence posture).

In some instances back pain may be related to damage or wear and tear to the inter-vertebral discs, muscular, tendon or ligament problems around the spine, or arthritis of the spine. Consultation with a GP is essential to identify potential causes and associated problems.

Signs and symptoms

Pain and discomfort in the low back with about 70 per cent of people reporting the experience of a dull and poorly localised referred pain to the legs and buttocks (Prodigy 2005*c*).

With appropriate management most people are pain-free and able to resume normal activities within three weeks. However, low back pain can vary in the intensity of pain experienced and is usually recurrent. Table 8.3 gives a list of questions that can be used in clinical practice to assess the severity of back pain.

Treatment

Medication

Medication is offered to relieve pain but cannot cure the condition. Paracetemol is usually first choice because side effects are low. NSAIDs (ibuprofen) are another option; however, long-term use is not recommended for lower back pain (as they can have adverse effects on other conditions, such as asthma, hypertension, etc.). A combination of both paracetemol and an NSAID, or codeine, is a further option. If pain relievers are ineffective, muscle relaxants (such as diazepam) can be offered, but only in short courses due to the risk of dependency.

Table 8.3	Questions used in clinical practice to assess the intensity of low back pain
Does back pain limit you?	*Standard limits*
Standing	Standing in one place for less than 30 minutes
Walking	Walking less than 30 minutes or 1–2 miles
Travelling by car or bus	Travelling less than 30 minutes
Socialising	Missing or curtailing of social activities (excluding sport)
Sleeping	Sleep disturbed by pain at least twice a week
Sex life	Sexual activity reduced or curtailed
Dressing	Help required to put on footwear

Adapted from Prodigy (2005*c*).

Functional activity

Getting back to normal activities as soon as possible is essential. The spine is designed to move, so bed rest does not promote recovery and can actually prolong pain and disability. During an episode of back pain, most activities need to be adapted and modified slightly, but the focus should be on getting on with life.

Positive mental attitude

Mental attitude has a strong influence on recovery. People who cope and get on with it and who are involved and committed to self-management of the condition (correcting posture, lifting correctly, etc.) usually recover much more quickly and have less long-term trouble. People who are frightened of the pain, fearful of further injury, who avoid activity and rest a lot hoping the pain will go away tend to suffer for longer and increase their risk of becoming more disabled by the condition.

Hot and cold treatments

Hot or cold treatments can be used to provide relief of pain and relax the muscles. Specific guidance from a physiotherapist should be sought and followed regarding the application of these treatments.

Massage

Gentle back-rubbing by a qualified practitioner (chiropractor, physiotherapist, osteopath) can help to soothe pain and relax muscles.

Relaxation and breathing

Stress and anxiety can contribute to back pain; therefore, learning to relax and using breathing to promote relaxation can assist with management. The Benson method of relaxation and relaxation breathing techniques (discussed in Chapter 7, section on stress-related disorders) is one useful method of relaxation.

Lifestyle

Assess the height and positioning of chairs and desks used at home or work and get up and move around and stretch regularly to avoid stiffening up. A back support can be used when driving, and when possible take regular breaks from driving and stretch out the body. Correct lifting should be practised when moving equipment and/or shopping. Use a wheel trolley for shopping. Sleep on a firm mattress. People who are overweight should aim to lose weight.

Posture awareness

Prolonged muscle imbalance by holding an incorrect posture will lead to increased muscle tension and tightness and may contribute to low back pain. In addition, poor posture, maintained and uncorrected for long periods of time, can also lead to permanent postural problems, for example lordosis (hollow back) can be a cause of low back pain, and also a hunched back posture (kyphosis) can contribute to the risk of falls in later life. Exercises to open and align posture can help to alleviate a build-up of muscular tension and can also enhance the functioning of inner organs (e.g. diaphragm). Pilates and yoga-based programmes focus on posture, mobility, flexibility and breathing. Learning to stand and sit correctly can be essential as part of self-management.

Exercise recommendations

There is no conclusive evidence base that makes recommendations for specific types of exercise or activity. The following are suggested for guidance.

Specific exercises to strengthen the abdominal and back muscles

- Abdominal hollowing;

Standing posture

- Stand with feet hip-width apart, feet parallel
- Distribute weight between heel bone, big toe and little toe (three-point weight distribution)
- Spread toes
- Align second toe with knee and hip
- Find neutral pelvic position (pubic bone and hip bones in line to ensure minimal forward or backward tilt of pelvis)
- Lengthen torso and neck
- Tighten the deeper abdominal muscles (so that the contraction can be maintained)
- Look forward – chin parallel to floor
- Shoulders relaxed and down
- Shoulder blades squeeze down
- Arms relaxed, hands by the side of body

Seated posture

- Sit on a chair with buttocks on the front one-third of the chair
- Align knees over ankles
- Place feet hip-width apart and parallel
- Distribute weight evenly between heel bone, big toe and little toe (three-point weight distribution)
- Spread toes
- Sit upright and lengthen spine
- Lift out of sitting bones to find neutral pelvic position (pubic bone and hip bones in line to ensure minimal forward or backward tilt of pelvis)
- Lengthen torso and neck
- Tighten the abdominals (so that the contraction can be maintained)
- Look forward – chin parallel to floor
- Shoulders to be relaxed and down
- Shoulder blades to squeeze down
- Keep arms relaxed, hands by side of chair

- Pilates-based abdominal exercises (lying heel slides, lying heel raises, lying knee raises, lying pelvic tilts, etc.);

- curl-ups and back extensions.

Gentle mobility of the spine

- Side bends (seated or standing);
- gentle rotations (seated or standing);
- Pilates-based mobility exercises for the spine (spine rotations, pelvic tilts, shoulder bridge, knee drops, etc.).

Flexibility exercises

- Hip flexors
- erector spinae
- hamstrings
- abductors
- obliques.

Core ball exercises

Maintaining correct seated posture while sitting on a core ball can assist strengthening the abdominals. Other gentle core ball exercises can be introduced:

- heel raises
- leg extensions
- pelvic tilts
- resistance exercises while seated on the ball (bicep curls, shoulder press, lateral raise, etc.).

Exercise in water

Exercise in water can be an effective exercise medium for people with low back pain. It provides support to the body-weight and may enable exercises to be performed for longer periods. The water provides a massaging effect, which can help to release muscle tension. Also, those who are fearful of hurting their backs can be assured of the additional support offered by exercising in water.

Correct posture and contraction of the abdominals to assist stability must be reinforced when exercising in water as buoyancy can affect both balance and posture.

Swimming may be performed, although care must be taken as some swimming strokes may aggravate low back pain.

See also table 8.4.

Exercise limitations

- Focus on correct posture and technique throughout.
- Ensure contraction of abdominals for all exercises.
- Avoid high impact.
- A postural assessment may be useful to identify and make provision for any muscle imbalances.

- Avoid heavy lifting.
- Avoid jerking and jarring movements.
- Avoid trunk exercises during episode of back pain (focus on abdominal hollowing).
- Avoid repetitive bending movements.
- Ensure correct lifting techniques.
- Avoid fast twisting or bending movements of the spine.
- Avoid double leg raising, straight leg sit-ups, straight leg dead lifting or other exercises that apply a heavy load to the spine.
- Avoid staying in one position for too long.
- Gentle mobility and stretching activities for the spine can be performed (Pilates).
- Contraindications for any other coexisting medical conditions should also be considered.

Table 8.4	Exercise guidelines, low back pain			
Training guidelines	Cardiovascular	Muscle strength	Flexibility	Functional
Frequency	3–5 days a week	2 days a week	5 days a week	2–3 days a week
Intensity	Dependent on current fitness and other conditions	Point of mild fatigue without loss of technique.	To point of mild tension	
Time	As above	<age 50: 8–12 reps, 1 set >age 50: 10–15 reps, 1 set	As long as is comfortable 3 reps of each stretch	
Type	Functional. Low impact. Brisk walk.	Abdominal and back extensor strength focus	Focus on flexibility of hip flexors and extensors and trunk muscles	Sit to stand. Correct lifting techniques. Correct posture.

Adapted from Durstine and Moore (2002: 218).

OBESITY

9

Obesity can be defined as a significant excess of body fat and is currently 'the major nutritional disorder facing westernised civilisations' (Waine 2002: 2). Obesity is often identified as providing a contributory risk to other, more serious health conditions, such as CHD, respiratory conditions, type 2 diabetes, joint problems (osteoarthritis), hypertension (high blood pressure), hyperlipidaemia (high cholesterol), stroke and some cancers (Waine 2002; Durstine and Moore 2003; McArdle, Katch and Katch 1991). It can also create an additional hazard and complications for individuals during pregnancy and/or for individuals undergoing surgery.

In addition to the physical and medical problems, the psychological impact of the condition should not be ignored: social discrimination (prejudice and bullying) and the struggle that many individuals face with experiences of dieting and trying to lose weight may contribute to feelings of distress, hopelessness, powerlessness, lowered self-esteem and depression. Obesity therefore has serious implications for an individual's health (physical, medical, mental, emotional and social) and overall well-being. Its contribution as a risk for other medical conditions means that it is fast becoming a major economic burden for the healthcare services in most developed countries (Waine 2002).

However, the paradox of obesity is that while the medical profession has been willing to recognise and treat the complications of obesity, it has been much less willing to treat obesity as a 'disease in its own right and devote it the time and attention that it deserves' (Waine 2002: 27).

The most common measure to define obesity is the BMI (body mass index). This calculates the individual's weight in kilograms (kg) and divides this by their height in metres squared (m^2).

Body mass index formula

$$BMI = \frac{Weight\ (kg)}{Height\ squared\ (m^2)}$$

For example: The calculation for an individual with a weight of 70 kg and a height of 1.75 m is

$$70 \div (1.75 \times 1.75) = 22.9\ BMI$$

One disadvantage of the BMI scale (see table 9.1) is that it does not distinguish the actual percentage of body fat, for example: a bodybuilder with low body fat and a high muscular weight might be classified as obese when calculating their weight in relation to their height (Brewer et al. 2003: 154).

Another key disadvantage of using the BMI scale is that it fails to distinguish between general obesity and truncal obesity (obesity in the trunk area of the body, which represents the apple-shaped rather than the pear-shaped body, or obesity around the hips and thighs). Truncal obesity is associated with other risk factors that include insulin resistance, hyperinsulinaemia, decreased glucose tolerance, decreased HDL (high-density lipoproteins) cholesterol, elevated LDL (low-density lipoproteins) cholesterol and triglycerides, and hypertension (high blood

Table 9.1	Body Mass Index	
BMI	Classed as	Health risk
Less than 18.5	Underweight	Some health risk
18.5 to 24.9	Ideal	Normal
25 to 29.9	Overweight	Moderate health risk
30 to 39.9	Obese	High health risk
40 and above	Very obese	Very high health risk

Table adapted from Prodigy (2003c).

pressure); this combination of symptoms is often known as 'syndrome X' (Waine 2002: 5). Thus, taking a weight measurement can give a further guide to risk. The waist circumference (see table 9.2) is a better indicator of health risk than BMI, especially in older people and people from South Asia.

Prevalence

More than half the UK adult population are heavier than recommended, with approximately two in five being overweight and one in five being obese. It is reported that over 6 million people are obese in the UK (Waine 2002: 1) and that the number of obese adults has almost tripled since 1980. It is also reported that women are the 'biggest weight gainers' with significant increases in body-weight occurring in the 25–34-year-old age group (McArdle, Katch and Katch 1991: 657). There has also been an increase of overweight children in the US in the last decade (Wallace 2003: 149), a trend that mirrors that of the UK, where the number of obese children has doubled since the early 1980s (Brewer et al. 2003: 158). Obesity is reaching epidemic proportions.

Cause

Most people will put on weight if the energy they put into their body (food and drink)

Table 9.2	Waist circumference	
Waist (men)	Waist (women)	Health risk
94 cm (37 inches)	80 cm (32 inches)	Moderate health risk
102 cm (40 inches)	88 cm (35 inches)	High health risk
Waist (Asian men)	Waist (Asian women)	
Greater than 90 cm (36 inches)	Greater than 80 cm (32 inches)	Increased health risk

Adapted from Prodigy (2003c); Diabetes UK (2004b).

exceeds their energy output (activity and exercise). However, there is no conclusive evidence as to what specifically causes obesity, and it is not simply a result of gluttony and over-eating, which is a common belief. There are a number of other factors that may contribute as causes for obesity, including:

- environmental and social factors (eating patterns, changes in technology, media, social class, education, marketing of food, food packaging, the diet industry, exercise and activity promotion, levels of inactivity, junk food, increased TV and computer games and/or computer-based work);

- genetic factors (having parents who are obese, which may be linked more with learning poor eating habits, although it may be that other genetic factors such as hormones and chemicals that control appetite may be faulty);

- physiological factors (metabolic rate, body type, fat cells);

- psychological factors (body image, eating patterns in relation to mood, trauma, comfort eating etc.);

- medical factors (less than one in 100 obese people have a medical cause, such as underactive thyroid. Some medications can contribute to weight gain, such as antidepressants and steroids).

These factors are to some extent intertwined, and each one will have an impact on another (Waine 2002: 12; McArdle, Katch and Katch 1991: 657; Prodigy 2005*f*).

However, the impact of decreasing inactivity in response to increasing reliance and dependence on technology (motorised transport, energy-sparing devices, lifts, escalators, video games, television and central heating) and changes in dietary habits over the last half-century (eating higher-fat diets and snacking,

which can reduce the conscious recognition of food being eaten and satiety) are recognised as being high contributory factors (Waine 2002: 13; Durstine and Moore 2003: 149).

Obesity often starts in childhood and this factor increases the prevalence of adult obesity at a ratio of approximately 3:1 in comparison to children of a normal body mass (McArdle, Katch and Katch 1991: 656).

Signs and symptoms

The major sign of obesity is obvious: obese people 'wear their problem for all to see at all times' (Waine 2002: 2). The psychological signs and symptoms, however, are usually much deeper and less observable. The impact of social prejudices and ignorance that begin in childhood in the playground can have long-lasting effects on the individual's self-esteem and self-worth.

Treatment

The aim of any treatment should be focused on managing rather than losing weight and measures of success need to be focused around effects of changes made to the individual's overall health and well-being, rather than changes to their body-weight per se.

Weight management and lifestyle interventions

Successful weight management and loss can be achieved through lifestyle interventions and changes that:

- Reduce energy intake (quantity and quality of food intake. For example: reducing higher-calorie, less nutritious food choices and increasing lower calorie and more nutritious food choices). NB: specific dietary advice must be offered by a qualified dietician.

- Increase energy output (frequency of activity and exercise).

- Interventions should fit with the individual's lifestyle and be easy for him or her to sustain.

- Offer regular support, to encourage the individual and identify the positive benefits of making changes.

An important discovery over recent years has been the effect of minor weight losses (5–10 per cent) on the reduction of other risk factors/ conditions such as high blood pressure, high cholesterol, diabetes, osteoarthritis, respiratory disorders, etc.

Waine (2002: 47) recommends a patient-centred approach that emphasises compassion and appropriate use of communication skills, intimacy and relational skills for helping individuals to manage obesity, which include being:

- empathetic as opposed to unconcerned;

- unbiased as opposed to judgemental;

- supportive as opposed to dismissive;

- accepting as opposed to fault-finding;

- optimistic as opposed to being sceptical.

The same relationship is essential between a personal trainer and client. Treating the individual with respect and an understanding and empathy towards the problems they face can impact the success of any weight-loss interventions. In particular, discussion regarding the individual's commitment is essential for assessing his or her readiness to make changes, which will ultimately impact the success of any interventions made. So too is the ability to establish realistic targets in relation to weight loss etc. The almost impossible goal of achieving their ideal body-weight should be avoided with obese individuals. A more realistic and achievable target of making small and progressive increases to their physical activity levels and small weight losses, with the emphasis being on the benefits of these losses on overall health, should be aimed at.

Hughes and Martin (1999) offer a range of suggestions for consideration when designing a weight-management programme. These include:

- raising the profile of exercise;

- support of GPs and health professionals to promote the benefits of exercise and activity;

- including a clinical psychologist in the team to assist with behaviour change;

- treating depression before making any attempt to start a weight-loss programme;

- assessing the individual's readiness and commitment to make changes;

- dietary recommendations that are aimed at the whole family, implemented gradually, and negotiated rather than imposed assists with compliance;

- the use of food diaries to assess current eating and drinking patterns is recommended;

- a combination of dietary advice and exercise is more effective than either intervention offered in isolation;

- group activities that are dependent on attendance at a facility to enhance support, motivation and monitoring of progress are more effective than attempting to go it alone (Waine 2002).

Counselling

Counselling can sometimes be useful for exploring the individual's relationship to food and eating patterns and choice of food. Being able to discuss struggles openly and honestly in a non-judgemental and supportive environment can increase the confidence of the individual and assist with their motivation towards making changes to improve health.

Specific strategies that can help the individual can also be explored. For example:

- keeping a food diary and becoming more conscious of eating behaviour;
- identifying healthier food options that are lower in fat and calories;
- recognising and managing stress or mood triggers that promote snacking or eating for comfort;
- eating more slowly;
- having smaller meals;
- discussing relapses and exploring strategies to overcome these;
- positive self-talk/affirmations.

Exercise recommendations

The actual exercise and activity recommendations suggested will be dependent on a number of factors, which include the individual's:

- level of obesity and its duration (how long have they been overweight/obese);
- current level of activity;
- age;
- other lifestyle factors that contribute to health (smoking etc.);
- other medical conditions (CHD, diabetes, depression);
- associated problems (joint pain, arthritis, high blood pressure, etc.);
- medication.

The benefits of exercise and activity are numerous and include: improved fitness, reduced risk of CHD, stimulation of fat oxidation, improved lipid profile, improved energy levels, decreased blood pressure, increased metabolic rate, improved psychological well-being, and potential appetite suppression (Waine 2002: 60).

An excellent starting point is to encourage the individual to become more active in their daily life. These smaller but more achievable activity goals will contribute to the individual's ability to tolerate other exercise and activity interventions. Examples include:

- walking more frequently to replace short journeys in the car or on public transport;
- walking for a short duration during work lunch breaks;
- walking up escalators or stairs rather than using lifts (even for a few floors, and progressing the number of floors climbed);
- doing the housework a little more vigorously and maybe more frequently;
- washing the car;
- taking up an active hobby (gardening, swimming, rambling, walking group);
- moving around more in the house (playing music and dancing, climbing stairs more frequently, etc.).

General mobility exercises Even when seated, short bouts of **chair-based** mobility, stretching and strengthening exercises can be performed. Again, these can be used to build the individual's tolerance for more sustained activity. They can also develop a habit and routine.

Cardiovascular activities are essential as part of a weight-management programme. The disadvantage for the obese individual and other individuals who may be aiming to lose weight is that the exercise needs to be sustained for a considerable duration and frequently to make an impact on body-weight. A pound of body fat is equivalent to 3,500 kilocalories and a significant amount of exercise would need to be performed to burn this number of calories. An obese individual is already carrying extra weight around with them and therefore may not be able to tolerate some activities for long durations. Activity needs to start off at a much lower intensity and for a shorter duration and progress steadily. This may make their progress slower, which can be disheartening. It is therefore essential to highlight all the positive steps and changes they make to self-manage their condition and highlight any positive changes to their health, even if this is quite simply feeling better about themselves. Each step the person makes towards increasing their activity throughout the day also needs to be acknowledged and validated as a personal contribution for improving their overall health, whether weight loss is or is not achieved.

Walking is an excellent low-impact activity. However, for the obese individual, long periods of time bearing their body-weight can be demanding (comparatively high intensity) and can place a lot of stress on the joints.

Low-weight-bearing cardiovascular machines such as exercise bikes and/or rowing machines may also be appropriate. However, the individual's ability to get on and off the machines will determine whether they can be used. Sensitivity is paramount as the individual will feel very self-conscious and these feelings will be heightened if the gym is busy and other people are watching. These factors may also affect the person's adherence to the programme. Tolerating feelings of shame and embarrassment is not easy and most people (obese or not) would choose to avoid these feelings! Therefore, environmental factors, such as the time of the session (gym-based programmes) and the empathy of the trainer are essential to promote the person's comfort and confidence.

Group exercise A specialist group exercise programme, which is much slower and lower in impact and intensity, may be appropriate. Once again, sensitivity to the individual's confidence should be considered, although group exercise can provide many social and motivational benefits. There is also evidence to show that obese people prefer to exercise with other obese people and that programmes that encourage the participation of friends and partners are recommended (Hughes and Martin 1999).

Exercise in water can be effective for obese people. First, it provides a support to the body-weight and may enable exercises to be performed for a longer duration without placing unnecessary or excessive stress on the joints (non-weight-bearing). Second, the support of the water will also enable exercises that could not be done safely on land (jogging, jumping, etc.) to be performed. As explained previously, being able to maintain and sustain performance of an activity for an extended duration is crucial for managing weight; therefore, exercise in water can contribute to this. Water also covers the body, so any self-conscious feelings pertaining to body image would be less apparent than if exercising in a more exposed environment (i.e. exercise studio or gym).

See also table 9.3.

Exercise limitations and considerations

- The individual's functional capacity will need to be considered as this will affect whether they are able to perform certain activities. For example: how easily can they get out of a chair (sit to stand)? Are they able to get on and off specific exercise equipment? Are they able to get up and down from the floor? Are they comfortable lying or sitting in certain positions? Does body bulk prevent them from performing certain exercises and stretches?

- Activity should be low impact and where possible non-weight-bearing.

Table 9.3	Exercise guidelines, obesity			
Training guidelines	Cardiovascular	Muscle strength	Flexibility	Functional
Frequency	5 days a week	2–3 days a week	Daily or 5 sessions a week	As comfortable to improve quality of life
Intensity	50–70% HRmax Monitor RPE and HR	Low resistance 40–50% of maximal voluntary contraction	To position of mild tension	Activity related to daily living
Time	Progress to 1 session of 40–60 min or 2 sessions of 20–30 min. Progress duration more than intensity. Activity can be accumulated if necessary.	1–3 sets 10–15 reps	To increase ROM	
Type	Large muscles and ideally non-weight-bearing. Swimming, cycling, exercise in water, walking. Low impact only. Vary activity to avoid overuse injury.	Circuit training approach. 8–10 different exercises	Stretching. Can include chair-based mobility and stretching. Controlled range of movement.	Walking. Sit to stand. Posture. Climbing stairs. Chair mobility.

Adapted from Durstine and Moore (2003: 212 and 29).

- The intensity will need to be comparatively low.
- The duration of the activity should be built progressively.
- Lower resistance must be used for any cardiovascular and muscular training as the body-weight is already adding to the resistance being moved!
- Body bulk may restrict range of motion.
- Speed of exercise should be slower to compensate for extra weight being carried.
- Music speed (if used) must be slower.
- Transitions and moving from one exercise to another will take longer.
- Becoming more active and building activity into daily life is an excellent starting point for developing a positive habit.
- Other medical conditions and medications must be taken into account and exercise guidelines and specific activities adapted accordingly.
- Maintaining levels of motivation by offering

support and encouragement and regular assessments can help adherence and management of any relapses.

- A sensitive and empathic approach from the instructor is essential.

- Community-based programmes may be more effective at attracting this group, as walking into a gym for the first time can be intimidating and most people would choose to avoid the feelings of humiliation and shame that can be triggered from past memories (e.g. playground taunting).

Exercising in an environment with other similar individuals (peers) can provide support and assist with building self-confidence.

- Keeping an activity and exercise diary can be useful to monitor activity.

- The use of a pedometer to measure steps taken in a day can also be a motivational tool and a way of monitoring progress.

- Encouraging the person to become involved in creating their own ways of becoming more active will promote adherence.

ENDOCRINE CONDITIONS

10

Diabetes

Diabetes comprises a group of disorders characterised by raised blood glucose levels (DoH 2001c). This section focuses on Type 1 and Type 2 diabetes.

Diabetes occurs when:

- there is a lack of the hormone insulin and/or
- the body is unable to respond to the action of insulin.

Insulin is produced by the pancreas and enables the cells of the body to use glucose, which is stored in the muscles and liver as glycogen. Glucose is broken down from the food we eat and is needed as a source of energy by most body tissues, including the brain and skeletal muscles. If there is insufficient insulin, no insulin, or the cells of the body are resistant to insulin action, the levels of blood glucose will increase. The cells of the body begin breaking down fat and protein as a source of energy and the kidneys produce extra urine to try and remove the excess glucose from the blood. This affects the way the body functions and results in hyperglycaemia (raised blood glucose levels) and the symptoms of diabetes (see box on page 100).

Insulin and glucagon are the two main hormones responsible for controlling blood glucose. Insulin is produced by beta cells in the pancreas, and glucagon is produced by alpha cells in the pancreas. In the absence of diabetes these two hormones work in partnership to maintain a healthy level of blood glucose, between 4 and 7 millimoles of glucose per litre of blood (mmol/l). When levels of blood glucose increase (e.g. after a meal) insulin levels rise to facilitate the uptake of glucose by the body cells. When blood glucose levels fall (e.g. skipping breakfast) glucagon is released. This converts glycogen in the liver back to glucose, resulting in increased blood glucose levels.

Type 1 diabetes

In Type 1 diabetes the pancreas no longer produces insulin. The insulin-producing beta cells in the pancreas have been destroyed by the body's immune system and there is no insulin to enable the blood glucose to move out of the bloodstream into the body cells. Glucose levels build up in the blood and are excreted in urine (DoH 2001c). Type 1 diabetes can develop at any age but usually develops at a much younger age than Type 2, often in childhood. Once developed, this condition is lifelong and the person will need to use insulin daily to survive. It cannot be cured, but can be controlled through daily insulin and eating a healthy diet. There is currently no evidence that exercise improves blood glucose control in Type 1 diabetes, as measured by HbA1c (AACPVR 2004). The main role of exercise in Type 1 diabetes is to modify risk factors for cardiovascular disease and improve overall health.

Type 2 diabetes

In Type 2 diabetes the beta cells in the pancreas are not able to produce enough insulin for the body's need, and/or the cells in the body become 'insulin resistant' and are unable to use insulin properly. Insulin resistance refers to how sensitive the organs and cells of the body are to the action of insulin. Type 2 usually develops later in life, although it is being increasingly diagnosed in children and adolescents. In the past it has been known as late-onset or non-insulin dependent diabetes mellitus (NIDDM); however, insulin may be part of an individual's treatment.

Unlike Type 1 diabetes, Type 2 is preventable and can be delayed by a change in lifestyle. Recent research has demonstrated that an increase in physical activity along with dietary changes can prevent or delay the onset of Type 2 diabetes in people at risk of the disease (ADA 2004).

Prevalence

Over 1.8 million people in the UK are diagnosed with diabetes, of which 1.5 million are diagnosed with Type 2. Another million people in the UK are thought to have undiagnosed Type 2 diabetes (Diabetes UK 2004*b*).

- Diabetes is increasing in all age groups
- Type 1 is increasing in children, particularly children under 5
- Type 2 diabetes is increasing across all groups, and particularly among people from black and ethnic minority groups
- Type 2 diabetes is more prevalent among less affluent populations and socially excluded groups such as prisoners, refugees and people with learning disabilities.

(DoH 2001*c.*)

Causes

Risk factors for **Type 1 diabetes** include:

- Genetic link: however, even if a person has genes associated with Type 1 diabetes they will not automatically develop diabetes.

- Environmental trigger: the disease may develop after an encounter with a trigger, possibly linked to certain viruses and chemicals, which causes the body's immune system to attack the beta cells in the pancreas (WHO 1999).

Risk factors for **Type 2 diabetes** include:

- family history of Type 2 diabetes;
- increasing age;
- obesity or central obesity;
- high blood pressure;
- lack of physical activity;
- *impaired glucose tolerance (IGT);
- *impaired fasting glycaemia (IFG).

(WHO 1999.)

*Impaired glucose tolerance (IGT) and impaired fasting glycaemia (IFG) indicate that the body is not processing glucose effectively. IGT is a stage of impaired glucose regulation and IFT is used to classify individuals who have fasting glucose levels above a normal range, but below those diagnostic of diabetes (Diabetes UK 2000). Both IGT and IFG are associated with an increased risk of developing diabetes and CVD (JBS 2005).

Signs and symptoms

In Type 2 diabetes the symptoms are mild or even absent; they develop gradually and people are often unaware of the development of the disease, which can remain undiagnosed for years. In Type 1 diabetes the symptoms are more obvious and usually develop over a few weeks.

Prevention of Type 2 Diabetes

There is strong evidence that both diet, physical activity and, where appropriate, drug therapy

---

Signs and symptoms of diabetes

Excessive thirst (polydypsia)
Excessive urination (polyuria)
Blurred vision
Unexplained weight loss (more evident in Type 1)
Recurrent infection such as thrush (evident in Type 2)
Tiredness

---

can prevent progression to diabetes and CVD (JBS 2005). In people with impaired glucose regulation a physical activity programme of at least 150 minutes a week of moderate to vigorous activity is recommended, alongside a healthy diet (ADA 2004).

Diagnosis

A GP will usually make a diagnosis based on symptoms, physical examination and the results of the following laboratory tests to measure blood glucose levels:

- fasting plasma glucose ≥6.0 mmol/l, or
- 2-hour plasma glucose ≥11.1 mmol/l following an oral glucose tolerance test (OGTT).

(Diabetes UK 2000; Joint British Societies *Guidelines* 2005.)

If it is difficult to tell whether the person has Type 1 or Type 2 diabetes the GP will carry out a test which checks for the presence of antibodies that attack the body or a substance called C-peptide (NICE 2004). The presence of antibodies or C-peptide indicates Type 1 diabetes.

HbA1c

Another blood test for diabetes is called haemoglobin A1c (HbA1c). This test is not used

as a diagnostic test; however, it is usually carried out on a 2–6-month basis and gives an idea of a client's overall average glucose control. HbA1c is formed when glucose in the blood 'sticks' to the haemoglobin in the red blood cells. The HbA1c measures the amount of glucose attached to the haemoglobin in the red blood cells. The Joint British Societies Guidelines (2005) recommend an HbA1c of ≤6.5 per cent.

Blood glucose levels

Ideally, blood glucose levels should be between 4 and 7 mmol/l before meals and <9 mmol/l two hours after meals (NICE 2004). The new Joint British Societies Guidelines recommend a slightly lower fasting or pre-prandial glucose value of 4.0–6.0 mmol/l as an optimal target for glycaemic control. Not everyone is able to maintain such a tight control and realistic goals for blood glucose management will need to be negotiated and agreed between the client and their health professional. It is important to maintain blood sugar levels as near to normal as possible to reduce the risk of developing complications of diabetes and the development of CVD.

Complications

The aim of diabetes treatment is to maintain blood glucose levels within appropriate margins, so that they are not too high (hyperglycaemia) or low (hypoglycaemia). Complications can be short- and long-term.

Hypoglycaemia

Hypoglycaemia is used to describe a low blood glucose level and is often called a 'hypo'. This refers to a blood glucose level below 4 mmol/l. However, everyone is different and people may experience hypoglycaemic symptoms at higher blood glucose levels or if there is a sudden drop in blood glucose levels. Hypoglycaemia occurs when there is too much insulin in the body, which may be caused by a number of factors including:

- a change in food intake, irregular or missed meals;
- the type and timing of medications such as insulin or insulin secretagogues;
- exercise;
- alcohol consumption.

It is important for the client and exercise professional to be aware of the signs and symptoms of hypoglycaemia and to know what to do in the event of a hypo (see table 10.1). Signs and symptoms can vary from person to person so ask the client to describe how hypoglycaemia affects her or him. Sometimes a carer or relative may be able to provide this information. A person on insulin therapy or insulin secretagogues such as sulphonylureas is at an increased risk of hypoglycaemia during or after exercise (See table 10.5, diabetic medications).

Hyperglycaemia

Hyperglycaemia refers to a raised blood glucose level above 10 mmols/l (Diabetes UK 2003*a*). The signs and symptoms of hyperglycaemia may include restlessness or nervousness initially, with more characteristic signs and symptoms such as thirst, fatigue and nausea developing over time. The following factors may lead to hyperglycaemia:

Insulin/diabetes medication A reduced dose or change in timing may cause blood

Table 10.1	Signs and symptoms of hypoglycaemia and hyperglycaemia
Hypoglycaemia	*Hyperglycaemia*
Trembling	Restlessness or nervousness
Sweating	Weakness
Anxiety	Increased thirst
Blurred vision	Dry mouth
Feeling faint	Decreased appetite
Feeling hungry	Nausea and vomiting
Paleness	Acetone breath
Mood change	
Confusion	
Elevated pulse	
Slurred speech	

Adapted from ACSM (2005).

glucose levels to rise. If a client is taking medication appropriately and is experiencing hyperglycaemia, a change in treatment may be required. A client who is managing diabetes with healthy eating and physical activity may need to begin taking tablets if they frequently experience raised blood glucose levels.

Change in physical activity A decrease in level of physical activity will result in a decreased use of glucose by the body and an increase in blood glucose levels. If a client is on insulin or insulin-like medication and their blood glucose levels are not well controlled, they are at an increased risk of hyperglycaemia during exercise.

Food intake An increase in the amount of food and a change in type of food will cause an increase in blood glucose level.

Stress/hormone change Stress hormones such as cortisol and adrenaline can affect the action of insulin and lead to a rise in blood glucose levels. Women may find that glucose levels are affected by the menstrual cycle and during the menopause (Walker and Rodgers 2004).

Illness During illness glycogen in the liver is converted to glucose. Increased levels of stress hormones will also be released, reducing the effectiveness of insulin. Both these actions result in an increased blood glucose level, requiring frequent monitoring.

Long-term hyperglycaemia increases the risk of diabetes-related complications.

Diabetic ketoacidosis (DKA)

This is caused by an inadequate concentration of insulin in the blood, which prevents the cells of the body taking up glucose and using it as a source of energy. The cells begin to rely on the body's fat reserves as a source of energy and the levels of blood glucose begin to rise. The by-products of fat metabolism are called ketones, which cause the blood to become more acidic.

This can lead to drowsiness and coma and is a potentially life-threatening condition. DKA is rare in people with Type 2 diabetes and is only likely to occur when there is another illness or infection (Diabetes UK 2003a).

Hyperosmolar non-ketotic acidosis (HONK)

This occurs in people with Type 2 diabetes who may be experiencing high blood glucose levels, often over 40 mmol/l. It develops over a few weeks and symptoms include frequent urination, increased thirst, nausea and, in later stages, drowsiness and gradual loss of consciousness. In people with Type 2 diabetes who are still producing some insulin, the acidic by-products associated with DKA are less likely to be produced. Hospital treatment is required to replace lost fluids and bring blood glucose levels down (Diabetes UK 2003a).

Long-term complications

If blood glucose levels remain elevated over a long period of time, the walls of the blood vessels become damaged. Microvascular damage affects the small arteries, veins and capillaries and can lead to complications including:

- Damage to nerves supplying the lower limbs, which can lead to loss of sensation, ulceration and lower limb amputation (peripheral neuropathy).

- Damage to the nerves can affect the involuntary function of the body including the cardiac, gastrointestinal and genitourinary systems (autonomic neuropathy).

- Damage to the small arteries of the retina at the back of the eye leads to visual impairment and blindness.

- Damage to the kidneys can lead to progressive kidney failure (nephropathy).

(DoH 2001.)

People with diabetes, especially people with Type 2 diabetes, are at an increased risk of macrovascular damage, which affects the walls of the larger blood vessels supplying the heart, brain and peripheries. This can lead to CVD including:

- coronary heart disease (angina and myocardial infarction)
- stroke and transient ischaemic attack (TIA)
- peripheral arterial disease, which can lead to pain on walking (claudication), leg and foot ulcers and limb amputation.

(DoH 2001c.)

The risk of dying from cardiovascular disease is doubled in men with diabetes and the risk of a heart attack is 50 per cent higher. For women with diabetes the risk of dying from cardiovascular disease is four times higher and the risk of a heart attack is 150 per cent higher (AACVPR 2004).

In order to reduce the likelihood of long-term complications it is important to try and keep the blood sugar level as normal as possible and to address other cardiovascular risk factors (high blood pressure, cholesterol, smoking, inactivity, obesity etc.).

Metabolic syndrome

The clustering of the risk factors is often found in people with central obesity and is referred to as the metabolic syndrome. An individual with metabolic syndrome is at an increased risk of cardiovascular disease. Risk factors include:

- blood pressure >135/80 mmHg;
- waist measurement more than 90 cm in women, or 100 cm in men; or 10 cm less in men and women with a South Asian background;
- low levels of high-density lipoprotein (HDL), the protective cholesterol;

- elevated triglycerides (type of blood lipids);
- insulin resistance;
- impaired glucose regulation including diabetes.

Weight reduction can play an important role in improving elements of the metabolic syndrome (NICE 2004b; JBS 2005).

Management of diabetes

According to the Joint British Societies Guidelines (2005), people with Type 1 and Type 2 diabetes are considered at high risk of CVD (≥20 per cent over 10 years) of developing atherosclerotic disease. In order to manage diabetes effectively and lessen the increased risk of CVD, a combination of lifestyle measures and drug therapies is recommended. Empowering people with diabetes is central to the National Service Framework (NSF) for diabetes (DoH 2001c). This is advocated through effective education, partnership with health professionals and shared decision making about health.

General goals for working with people with diabetes

- Maintain blood glucose levels within an appropriate range.
- Support lifestyle change to help control diabetes and reduce the long-term complications associated with diabetes.
- Provide individualised, culturally appropriate diabetes-specific advice about exercise and physical activity.
- Reduce the risk of cardiovascular disease.

People with long-term conditions such as diabetes are more likely to get anxious and depressed, which can have a detrimental affect on the management of their diabetes (NICE 2004). Education can play an important role in managing diabetes, and help to improve knowledge, blood glucose control, weight and dietary management, physical activity and psychological well-being (DoH 2001*c*). Education is particularly effective when it is tailored to the needs of the individual and addresses attitudes, skills and knowledge.

Lifestyle measures include:

- stopping smoking
- eating more healthily
- increasing levels of physical activity
- achieving optimal weight and weight distribution.

Risk factor targets

Blood pressure In people with diabetes a BP target of <130 mmHg systolic and <80 mmHg diastolic is recommended. People with diabetes and elevated blood pressure will be offered antihypertensive medication (See table 12.7).

Blood glucose control Tight control of glycaemia is recommended:

- fasting or preprandial glucose of 4–6.0 mmol/l, and
- HbA1c < 6.5 per cent.

(JBS, 2005.)

Cholesterol The optimal target for total cholesterol is <4.0 mmol/l *and* low-density lipoprotein (LDL) cholesterol < 2.0 mmol/l, or a 25 per cent reduction in total cholesterol *and* a 30 per cent reduction in LDL cholesterol, whichever achieves the lowest value (JBS 2005). Cholesterol-lowering medication called statins will be recommended to improve cholesterol levels (JBS 2005; NICE 2004*b*). (See table 12.7.) Statins are recommended for all people with diabetes (Type 1 and 2) over the

age of 40 and for some younger people with diabetes who have diabetic complications or an increased risk of CVD.

Antithrombotic therapy Aspirin is recommended for some people with diabetes to reduce the risk of CVD (NICE 2004*b*). If aspirin is not appropriate, an alternative, clopidogrel, might be prescribed. (Refer to table 12.7.)

Exercise recommendations

The aim of an exercise programme is to maximise the benefits of physical activity and minimise the complications associated with diabetes. The American College of Sports Medicine (2005*a*) recommends that people with diabetes planning moderate- to high-intensity activity should undergo a graded exercise test if the following criteria apply:

- age ≥ 35;
- Type 2 diabetes >10 years duration;
- Type 1 diabetes >15 years duration;
- presence of any additional risk factor for cardiovascular disease;
- presence of any microvascular disease (retinopathy or nephropathy);
- peripheral vascular disease;
- autonomic neuropathy.

This would provide useful information; however, a graded exercise test is not standard practice in the UK. In the absence of a graded exercise test it is advisable for a client with diabetes to be assessed by their GP prior to increasing their levels of physical activity. This should include taking a medical history and a comprehensive physical examination especially in relation to diabetic complications affecting the heart and circulatory system, eyes, kidneys, feet and nervous system. This will ensure that the diabetes is well controlled and will identify any conditions that require referral to a specialist and/or a specific exercise prescription.

Benefits of exercise

Exercise can benefit insulin sensitivity, hypertension, and blood lipid control. It has an important role in reducing the risk of cardiovascular disease and improving overall health and well-being. In many cases, Type 2 diabetes can be effectively managed by lifestyle measures such as a healthy diet, weight loss and increasing levels of physical activity. Exercise has a role in improving self-efficacy, psychological well-being and stress management, which can contribute to better self-management and improved quality of life (Diabetes UK 2003b).

Key considerations before starting an exercise programme

- Client is assessed by GP, is stable and exhibits no contraindications to exercise.
- Diabetes is well controlled.
- Client is taught about appropriate footwear and ongoing foot care.
- Client is aware of the effect of activity on blood glucose levels (hypoglycaemia and hyperglycaemia).
- Client knows the signs and symptoms of hypoglycaemia and knows what action to take.
- Client is able to self-monitor blood glucose levels.
- Client has discussed treatment changes such as adjusting insulin dosage and/or carbohydrate intake prior to exercise and for 24 hours afterwards.

NB: Refer also to Chapter 4 for other contraindications to exercise, and Chapter 6 for management of hypoglycaemia and hyperglycaemia in the exercise environment.

General guidelines for management of blood sugar levels before exercise

Monitoring blood glucose before exercise will ensure that it is safe to exercise and minimise the risk of worsening hyperglycaemia and hypoglycaemia in clients on insulin or oral hypoglycaemic agents. It important to take into account other factors including:

- intensity and duration of the activity;
- timing and dose of medication;
- time of the exercise session;
- type of insulin or oral medication;
- timing of last meal;
- individual response.

The general guidelines below are based on current UK (Diabetes UK), American College of Sports Medicine (2005) and American Diabetes Association (2004) recommendations. There are differences between these recommendations and it is important to work within guidelines that are developed locally between diabetes specialists and physical activity providers. Much of this advice on glucose monitoring is specific to clients on insulin or insulin secretagogues (see 'Medication for diabetes' later in this chapter). It is important to remember that every individual has a different metabolic response to exercise. Appropriate monitoring and observation will help you learn more about your client's response to exercise, develop an individualised programme and enable the client to exercise more safely and effectively.

In America, milligrams per decilitre (mg/dl) are used to measure glucose levels, which can make it confusing when trying to compare with UK or European guidelines. To convert mmol/l of glucose to mg/dl, multiply by 18. To convert mg/dl of glucose to mmol/l, divide by 18 or multiply by 0.055 (see table 10.2).

Table 10.2	Conversion chart
mg/dl	*mmol/l*
80	4.4
100	5.5
240	13.2
250	13.75
300	16.5

Some of the recommendations below may be more appropriate to clinical settings, especially where ketone testing is advised.

Pre-activity screening If blood glucose level < 5.5 mmol/l (< 100 mg/dl) the client will need to eat some additional carbohydrate (ACSM 2005). The amount of carbohydrate needed will depend on the intensity and duration of the planned exercise. Check that blood glucose levels have increased before starting to exercise and that the client has no symptoms of hypoglycaemia. These recommendations are appropriate for individuals on insulin and/or insulin secretagogues. Hypoglycaemia is rare in individuals who are not on insulin or insulin secretagogues and supplementary carbohydrate is not generally necessary (ADA 2004).

If blood glucose levels are >13 mmol/l (Diabetes UK 2004*a*), discuss possible reasons for blood glucose level and ask client to test for ketones in urine. Test strips are available from GP. If ketone levels are elevated, refer client to GP.

Do not exercise if:

- Blood glucose level is >13 mmol/l and ketone testing is inappropriate or not possible.
- Blood glucose level is >13 mmol/l with ketones (Diabetes UK 2004*a*).

The American Diabetes Association (2004) suggests that this may be over-cautious for a person with Type 2 diabetes, especially if the person has recently eaten. If the person feels well and ketones are negative, it may not be necessary to postpone low to moderate exercise based simply on hyperglycaemia. However, it is important to encourage good glycaemic control and the aim is to exercise in the presence of optimal glycaemic control.

Exercise with caution if:

- Blood glucose level is >13 mmol/l without ketones, as there may not be enough insulin to mobilise sufficient glucose for exercise (Diabetes UK 2004).

Practical recommendations for community exercise setting

Blood glucose levels should be in the range of 5.5–13 mmol/l (Diabetes UK 2004*a*). Some people are more cautious and recommend postponing exercise for clients on insulin when glucose levels are >200 mg/dl, which is approximately equivalent to 11 mmol/l (Russell and Sherman 1999).

If you have any concerns about a client exercising you can let him or her begin the session and ask them to monitor his or her blood glucose during exercise. If the blood glucose levels stay the same or begin to rise, you can ask the client to stop exercising and take appropriate action.

During exercise

If activity is vigorous or lasts more than an hour the client may need to check if blood glucose levels have fallen during activity and consume additional carbohydrate, e.g. a sugary drink or carbohydrate snack.

After exercise

Check blood glucose level after exercise to identify if food intake is necessary.

If the client feels shaky, anxious, confused or has a low blood glucose level, encourage her or him to have a fast-acting snack, followed by a sandwich or piece of fruit. A client with Type 2 diabetes who is not on insulin therapy or insulin secretagogues is unlikely to have a hypo-glycaemic episode during exercise, but may need to have something to eat after exercise.

An individual who has a tendency towards hypoglycaemia may need to adjust her or his treatment by reducing the dose of insulin or insulin secretagogue or increasing carbohydrate intake before or during exercise. If you have any concerns about the client's diabetes control, refer her or him to the GP or specialist diabetes team.

Guidelines for exercise

The guidelines for Type 1 diabetes are very similar to those for apparently healthy adults; however, the guidelines for people with Type 2 diabetes are more closely aligned to those for obesity, with a focus on increased caloric expenditure (ACSM 2005). There are differences between the ACSM (2005) and the American Diabetes Association (2004) guidelines based on emerging research. These are highlighted below.

Cardiovascular

The main aim of cardiovascular exercise is to improve glycaemic control, reduce the risk of cardiovascular disease and help with weight loss or weight maintenance. Clients with Type 2 diabetes can be encouraged to accumulate a minimum of 1,000 kcal a week of physical activity. If weight loss is a goal an additional caloric expenditure of ≥ 2000 kcal per week may be required (ACSM 2005). Daily exercise may be required to meet this challenge. The American Diabetes Association (2004) recommends the following:

- moderate intensity activity (40–60 per cent VO_2max, 50–70 per cent HRmax) for at least 150 minutes per week; and/or
- vigorous intensity activity (>60 per cent of VO_2max or >70 per cent of HRmax) for at least 90 minutes;
- distribute physical activity over at least three days a week, with no more than two consecutive days without physical activity.

The duration and intensity of the activity will depend on the specific goals of the individual and co-morbidities. In the absence of exercise stress testing and in a community setting, it may be more appropriate to exercise at moderate levels of intensity.

Muscular strength

There is a growing body of evidence for the value of resistance training in Type 2 diabetes (ADA 2004). The ACSM (2005) recommend a low-resistance (40–60 per cent 1RM) strength programme for clients with diabetes. The American Diabetes Association (2004) previously endorsed a similar programme; however, in the light of new research they currently recommend a moderate intensity (60–80 per cent 1RM) strength-training programme. A conservative approach is suggested, beginning with one set of 10–15 repetitions 2–3 times a week at a moderate intensity, and progressing to three sets of 8–10 repetitions at a weight that cannot be lifted more than 8–10 times (8–10 1RM). Although one set is sufficient for building strength, three sets produce greater metabolic benefits for people with Type 2 diabetes. It is important to consider co-morbidities when recommending higher-intensity resistance training, as it may be inappropriate or contraindicated for people with hypertension, retinopathy or joint problems.

Flexibility

There are no diabetes-specific guidelines for flexibility. The guidelines included reflect guidelines for the general population.

See also table 10.3.

Exercise limitations and considerations

- *Encourage clients to measure their blood glucose levels before and after exercise. If the exercise lasts for more than one hour, monitor blood glucose levels during the session as well.

- *Clients should reduce their insulin dose for planned activity/exercise. This will involve some degree of experimenting, as everyone responds differently; it will also depend on the duration and intensity of the activity and the dose and timing of insulin. Advise clients to discuss this with their diabetes team or healthcare professional.

- Plan exercise 1–2 hours after meals. It is best to avoid exercising during the peak insulin

Table 10.3	Summary of exercise guidelines for Type 2 diabetes		
Training guidelines	Cardiovascular	Muscle strength	Flexibility
Frequency	>3 days a week depending on goals. Clients on insulin and/or clients who are trying to lose weight may need to exercise daily.	2 (non-consecutive) days per week (ACSM 2005). 2–3 days per week (ADA 2004).	Minimum 2–3 days per week. Ideally 5–7 days a week.
Intensity	Moderate intensity activity (50–70% HRmax	40–60% 1RM (ACSM 2005) 8–10 1RM (ADA 2004) i.e. a weight that cannot be lifted more than 8–10 times.	To the point of tightness, below the point of discomfort.
Time	20–60 minutes depending on goal.	1 set of exercise 10–15 reps (ACSM 2005). Build up to 3 sets of 8–10 reps (ADA 2004).	Hold each stretch 15–30 seconds, 2–4 repetitions for each stretch.
Type	Walking, cycling, swimming, rowing. Weight bearing or non-weight bearing depending on presence of diabetic complications.	8–10 muscle groups that train major muscle groups. Target specific areas of weakness.	Static stretches
Functional	Balance and coordination activities for clients at risk of falls (peripheral neuropathy).		

ACSM (2005); ADA (2004).

action as this, combined with exercise, increases the risk of hypoglycaemia.

- *Use injection sites away from areas of the body predominantly used during exercise. The abdomen is the preferred site.

- *Clients should always carry fast-acting carbo-hydrate snacks or drinks when exercising.

- *Delayed hypoglycaemia can occur up to 36 hours after intense exercise as the muscles refuel. Make adjustments to the timing of exercise or encourage clients to eat a snack before going to bed. This is important if the client exercises in the evening, as there is an increased risk of nocturnal hypoglycaemia.

- Clients with Type 2 diabetes who are not on insulin or suphonylureas are unlikely to have a hypo; however, they may need to eat soon after exercise.

- Certain medications can mask or increase the risk of hypoglycaemia, including beta-blockers, calcium channel blockers and diuretics.

- Clients should drink plenty of water before, during and after activity to avoid dehydration.

- Alcohol inhibits glucose production, causing a hypoglycaemic effect. This hypoglycaemic effect can last up to 24 hours.

- Encourage daily foot inspection and remind clients to inform you about any changes such as blisters or inflammation.

*Specific considerations for people on insulin or insulin secretagogues, who are more at risk of hypoglycaemia during exercise or after exercise.

(Adapted from ACSM 2005; AACVPR 2004; NICE 2004.)

See also table 10.4.

Diabetes and Ramadan

Ramadan is a holy month in Islam, and all healthy adult Muslims are expected to fast. Ramadan lasts between 29 and 30 days and Muslims abstain from eating, drinking, smoking or using oral medications between dawn (*Suhur*) and sunset (*Iftar*). The Koran exempts people with medical conditions; however, many people with diabetes decide to fast, often against the advice of the medical profession. Fasting can lead to complications such as hypoglycaemia, hyperglycaemia, diabetic ketoacidosis and dehydration. The level of risk will depend on the type of diabetes, level of control and ability to self-manage. People with diabetes who decide to fast should have a pre-Ramadan assessment and educational counselling to reduce the risks (American Diabetes Association 2005). Normal levels of physical activity can be maintained; however, excessive physical activity or exercise may increase the risk of hypoglycaemia, especially in the hours before breaking the fast at sunset. People with poorly controlled Type 1 diabetes may be at an increased risk of hyperglycaemia. The daily prayers after sunset (*Tarawaih*) can be considered as part of the person's daily physical activity. If your client wants to continue his/her exercise programme during Ramadan, it is important to work closely with the client and the diabetes team to ensure that diabetes is well managed and the exercise programme adapted to minimise risk.

Medication for diabetes

Some people with Type 2 diabetes may be able to maintain target blood glucose levels by making lifestyle changes such as losing weight and increasing physical activity levels. If glucose levels remain high, medication is usually advised (see table 10.5) in addition to the recommended lifestyle changes. If, over time, blood glucose start to rise, additional medication may be prescribed. The main groups include:

- **Biguanide** Usually prescribed for someone who is overweight and unable to control blood glucose adequately through lifestyle intervention alone.

Table 10.4	Recommendations and precautions for clients with diabetic complications
Complications	Recommendations/precautions
Retinopathy (*Proliferate and severe stages: when the normal retinal blood vessels become obstructed new abnormal vessels begin to grow or proliferate. These blood vessels are weak and prone to bleeding.)	**Avoid** Contact sports. Activities that raise blood pressure (high-intensity resistance training or aerobic activity. Activities that lower the head (some yoga positions), jar the head or involve breath-holding or straining. **Recommendation** Have regular eye examinations to establish level and progression of retinopathy. Keep to low-level intensity training.
Peripheral neuropathy	**Precautions** Loss of protective sensation in the feet could increase the likelihood of musculoskeletal and orthopaedic injuries. Avoid prolonged weight-bearing activities (stepping, walking or high-impact activities). Loss of sensation can lead to problems with balance and increased risk of falls, so provide support where appropriate and include specific balance exercises. **Recommendation** Perform non-weight-bearing exercises such as chair-based exercise, cycling, rowing and water-based exercise (unless ulcers present), and/or Circuit-based programme – combining cycling, rowing, chair-based exercises and limited weight-bearing activities. Wear cushioned shoes.
Autonomic neuropathy	**Precautions** There may be abnormal heart rate and blood pressure at rest and in response to exercise. Risk of cardiac dysfunction, hypoglycaemia, silent ischaemia and dehydration is increased. **Recommendations** Avoid rapid changes in body position and be aware of post-exercise orthostatic hypotension. Ensure adequate hydration. Use RPE, alongside careful monitoring. May require clinical setting for exercise.
Nephropathy	**Avoid** Avoid activity that increases blood pressure (high-intensity aerobic or resistance training, breath-holding). **Recommendation** Perform low-intensity activity aerobic and resistance training. Ensure adequate hydration.

Type 2: adapted from ACSM (2005); AACVPR (2004).

- **Insulin secretagogues** Increase insulin secretion and include sulphonylureas and prandial glucose regulators (nateglinide and repaglinide). There is a risk of hypoglycaemia with these medications.
- **Thiazolidinediones (glitazones)** Increase the amount of glucose taken up from the blood and reduce blood glucose levels. Prescribed for people who can't take metformin and insulin secretagogues.
- **Alpha glucosidase inhibitor** Delays the absorption of carbohydrate, reducing the rise in glucose levels that occurs after eating. Prescribed for people who are unable to use other oral drugs.
- **Insulin** May be used for people with Type 2 diabetes, to control blood glucose levels if other medications have not been effective.
- **Orlistat** This may be prescribed for people with Type 2 diabetes who are overweight, as part of a plan to lose weight and maintain blood glucose levels.

(Diabetes UK 2005.)

Type 1

People with Type 1 diabetes need to take insulin every day to manage their blood glucose. There are numerous types of insulin and it is important for people to find the type and pattern of insulin that suits their lifestyle and helps them manage their glucose levels effectively.

Insulin

The goal of insulin treatment is to supply the body with the insulin it lacks and to mimic the normal pattern of insulin release throughout the day. There are a number of different types of insulin, including:

- **Rapid-acting insulin analogues** A synthetic form of insulin that aims to work like normal insulin to cope with a meal. The effects are short-lasting.
- **Short acting** Work more slowly, with the effect lasting up to eight hours.
- **Intermediate acting** Have an effect that can last through the night.
- **Long-acting** Can last for a longer period, e.g. a whole day.
- **Biphasic insulin** A mixture of rapid- or short-acting and intermediate-acting insulin (NICE 2004).

These work for different lengths of time in the body and are often prescribed in different combinations to control blood glucose levels adequately. The prescribed type and combination of insulin is called a regimen. Generally, an insulin regimen will provide a background level of insulin with additional boosts during the day. The insulin regimen may need to be adjusted to meet the needs of changes such as increasing levels of physical activity, eating patterns or periods of feeling unwell. In the longer term, changes in health and lifestyle may necessitate a change in regimen. As an exercise specialist it is appropriate to give your client general advice about physical activity and insulin treatment; however, it is important to ask your client to discuss any proposed change in physical activity and insulin regimen with his or her GP or specialist diabetes health professional. Insulin cannot be taken as a tablet because it would be digested by the body before getting into the blood supply, so it has to be injected (NICE 2004).

Table 10.5	Summary of medications for Type 2 diabetes (not including insulin) NICE 2002; Prodigy 2005; Diabetes UK 2005)		
Drug	Action	Side effects	Exercise implications/comments
Sulphonylureas *Glibenclamide Glimepiride Gliclazide*	Stimulates pancreas to produce more insulin. Helps insulin work more effectively.	Can cause weight gain. Nausea, mild diarrhoea and constipation are uncommon side effects. Possibility of hypoglycaemia.	Possibility of hypoglycaemia. Follow guidelines for people on insulin therapy.
Biguanide *Metformin*	Lowers blood glucose level by decreasing the. amount of glucose the liver releases into the bloodstream.	Can cause mild diarrhoea and sickness when first started. Less likely to cause weight gain than other glucose-lowering medications. Not prescribed for people with kidney problems.	None known.
Thiazolidinediones *Pioglitazone Rosiglitazone*	Increases sensitivity of cells to insulin, thereby increasing uptake of glucose into the cells.	Weight gain, oedema (fluid retention). Slight risk of liver damage, therefore a blood test to check on liver function is carried out before taking these medications. This is rechecked on a regular basis. Hypoglycaemia possible, but uncommon.	Hypoglycaemia possible, but uncommon.
Prandial glucose regulator *Nateglinide and repaglinide*	Similar action to sulphonylureas. Rapid onset and short duration of action.	Weight gain and hypoglycaemia.	Hypoglycaemia possible, but lower risk than sulphonylureas.
Alpha glucosidase inhibitor *Acarbose*	Delays absorption of carbohydrate from the intestine. Can prevent blood glucose peaks after meals.	Wind, bloating and diarrhoea.	None known.

RESPIRATORY DISORDERS

11

Respiratory disorders can be divided into restrictive and obstructive disease.

Restrictive disease is characterised by reduced lung volume as a result of a wide range of disorders that affect the thorax or the lung parenchyma (lung tissue) such as ankylosing spondylitis, kyphoscoliosis, spinal cord injury, and pulmonary fibrosis.

Obstructive disease is characterised by increased airway obstruction and expiratory resistance. Airway obstruction is caused by conditions such as bronchitis, emphysema and asthma. Chronic obstructive pulmonary disease (COPD) is the umbrella term for chronic bronchitis and emphysema; however, COPD can also include chronic asthma.

This section will focus on COPD (emphysema and bronchitis) and asthma, and the role of exercise within these conditions.

Chronic obstructive pulmonary disease

'COPD is a chronic disabling disease in which the patient's airways and sometimes the lungs themselves have become obstructed, causing persistent and progressive damage which can greatly impair the ability to lead a normal life. The disease is predominantly caused by smoking and nearly all sufferers are over 35' (NICE 2004).

Chronic bronchitis

In chronic bronchitis the bronchi (airways) become irritated or inflamed, often in response to cigarette smoking. As a result of the inflammation mucous starts to build up in excessive amounts, causing a chronic productive cough. The bronchi become narrowed, obstructing the flow of air in and out of the lungs. These symptoms may lead to breathlessness (dyspnoea).

Emphysema

This is caused by permanent enlargement and damage of the alveoli or air sacs in the lungs. This makes them much less efficient in transferring the gases of respiration between the lungs and the bloodstream, often leading to lower oxygen levels in the blood. The damage to the walls of the alveoli reduces the elastic recoil of the lungs. This means that expiration becomes an active rather than a passive action. It becomes difficult to push air out of the lungs and air becomes trapped, causing hyperinflation of the lungs. The muscles surrounding the bronchi can also become tighter, which results in bronchospasm, or 'wheeze', as air is squeezed through the airways.

Causes

Smoking is the main risk factor for the development of COPD; however, genetic and environmental factors may play a part in the development of the disease, such as:

- genetics;
- gender;
- occupation – where there is long-term exposure to certain types of dust or chemicals;

- environmental pollution (indoor air pollution in poorly ventilated living conditions and outdoor air pollution);
- socio-economic status;
- passive smoking also contributes to respiratory symptoms and COPD;
- respiratory infections in early childhood are associated with reduced lung function and respiratory conditions in adulthood.

(GOLD 2005; ATS and ERS 2005.)

Prevalence

'COPD is the leading cause of morbidity and mortality worldwide and results in an economic and social burden that is both substantial and increasing' (ATS and ERS, 2005).

Nearly 900,000 people in England and Wales are diagnosed as having COPD. A further 450,000 may be living with undiagnosed COPD (NICE 2004). More than 250,000 people die each year from its end stages, with ill health contributing to a poor quality of life before they die (Prodigy 2004).

Signs and symptoms

COPD affects people in different ways; however, the main symptoms are:

- a productive cough (coughing up sputum/phlegm);
- a chronic cough (intermittent or every day);
- breathlessness that is:
  - worse over time
  - present every day
  - worse on exercise
  - worse during respiratory infections;
- an increase in chestiness or wheezing during cold weather;

- peripheral muscle weakness;
- fatigue.

(NICE 2004; GOLD 2005.)

A cough is usually the first symptom. Initially the cough will come and go, but over time the cough becomes more persistent (chronic). As the airways become more damaged they produce more mucous, and phlegm may be coughed up every day. This occurs mainly with bronchitis, but not emphysema.

Breathlessness (dyspnoea) is one of the main symptoms of COPD and is the term used to describe subjective feelings of breathing discomfort. Dyspnoea may occur if the respiratory muscles have to work harder than expected to produce a given amount of ventilation (Ambrosino and Scano 2004). Dyspnoea is one of the most debilitating and frightening symptoms of COPD and often leads to people avoiding any activities that might make them breathless. Many people with COPD can get stuck in a cycle of inactivity, which leads to a decrease in fitness and functional capacity. This in turn results in an increase in respiratory effort and breathlessness to carry out daily activities. Before a diagnosis of COPD has been made, many people experience breathlessness that limits activity involving heavy exertion. They often associate this with getting old and don't access health services until their condition deteriorates further. Activities of daily living and recreational activities become increasingly difficult and uncomfortable as the disease progresses. This cycle of inactivity can lead to isolation, anxiety and depression. Patients can benefit from learning techniques to relieve feelings of breathlessness. Learning to manage breathlessness is an important part of a pulmonary rehabilitation programme as it can give people more control over their condition, and contributes to an improved quality of life.

Table 11.1	Differences between COPD and asthma		
		COPD	Asthma
Smoker or ex-smoker		Nearly all	Possibly
Symptoms under age of 35		Rare	Common
Chronic productive cough		Common	Uncommon
Breathlessness		Persistent and progressive	Variable
Night-waking with breathlessness and/or wheeze		Uncommon	Common
Significant diurnal or day-to-day variability of symptoms		Uncommon	Common

NICE (2004).

Diagnosis

A diagnosis will be made based on a history of the patient's symptoms and the results of several tests:

- over 35 with a risk factor (generally smoking);
- history of chronic progressive symptoms such as a cough, wheeze or breathlessness;
- airway obstruction confirmed through use of spirometry;
- no clinical features of asthma. Table 11.1 highlights the differences between COPD and asthma.

A full assessment by a GP should include: spirometry, breathlessness, weight loss and frequency of exacerbations (NICE 2004).

Spirometry

A device called a spirometer is used to measure how well the lungs are working and identify any reduction in expiratory flow. Two measurements are taken: the forced expiratory volume in one second (FEV1) and the forced vital capacity (FVC).

- FEV1 (forced expiratory volume in 1 second) measures the maximum amount of air that someone can force out of the lungs in one second.
- FVC (forced vital capacity) measures the total amount of air that someone can force out of his or her lungs after a maximal inspiration.
- The FEV1/FVC ratio is the FEV1 divided by the FVC.

A FEV1 (forced expiratory volume in 1 second) of less than 80 per cent predicted and a FEV1/FVC ratio of less than 70 per cent (0.7) indicates airway obstruction and the possibility of COPD. FEV1 is influenced by age, gender and ethnicity and is expressed as a percentage of a normal predicted value. There is a gradual decrease in both these measurements with age; however, smoking significantly accelerates this process and stopping smoking causes the decline in lung function to return to a 'normal' rate (GOLD 2005).

Spirometry is required to make a diagnosis of COPD, and can be used to monitor the progression of the disease. Table 11.2 indicates FEV1 values and the severity of airflow obstruction.

Table 11.2	Severity of airflow obstruction
Severity of airflow obstruction	FEV1 % predicted
Mild	50–80
Moderate	30–49
Severe	<30

Nice (2004).

Breathlessness (dyspnoea)

The level of dyspnoea does not necessarily relate to the severity of airway obstruction and it is possible for someone to have mild airway obstruction and severe dyspnoea. Dyspnoea is a subjective sensation of the severity of breathing discomfort experienced; however, it can be quantified using a scale. The effect of breathlessness on functional status or daily activities can be measured by using the Medical Research Council dyspnoea scale (Table 11.3).

Weight loss

Weight loss due to inadequate dietary intake, increased resting energy expenditure and muscle wasting may lead to a low body mass index (BMI) in patients with COPD. If a person's BMI is below the normal range of 20–24 they may need to supplement their diet to increase their calorie intake. This is especially relevant if the person is increasing their energy expenditure through increased physical activity.

Exacerbations

Managing exacerbations is one of the key priorities of the NICE COPD guidelines (2004). An exacerbation may occur from time to time, with a worsening of symptoms such as breathlessness, cough and volume of sputum. Symptoms may also include a cold or sore throat, reduced exercise tolerance, fluid retention and fatigue. An exacerbation can be infectious or non-infectious (ATS and ERS 2005). It is important that patients are aware of the symptoms of an exacerbation and know how to respond promptly. Appropriate use of inhaled corticosteroids, bronchodilators and an annual influenza vaccination should reduce the frequency of exacerbations. An

Table 11.3	Medical Research Council (MRC) dyspnoea scale
Grade	Degree of breathlessness related to activities
1	Not troubled by breathlessness except on strenuous exercise
2	Short of breath when hurrying or walking up a slight hill
3	Walks slower than contemporaries on the level because of breathlessness, or has to stop for breath when walking at own pace
4	Stops for breath after walking about 100 m or after a few minutes on the level
5	Too breathless to leave the house, or breathless when dressing or undressing

exacerbation will usually require a change in medications.

Additional tests used to diagnose COPD

- Chest X-ray to rule out any other causes of the symptoms.
- Blood test to find out if symptoms are caused by anaemia.
- Breathing tests using a peak flow meter to check for asthma; this will be carried out at different times of the day, over several days.
- A blood test for alpha-1 antritrypsin, an enzyme that protects the lungs from harmful substances such as cigarette smoke; this test is more likely to be used if a person is under the age of 40 and has never smoked.
- A TLCO (transfer factor for carbon dioxide) test to assess the lungs' ability to transfer oxygen to the bloodstream; this will usually be carried out if the results of a spirometer test are especially low.
- A computed tomography (CT) scan for a more detailed assessment of the condition of the lungs.
- An (ECG) electrocardiogram and/or an echocardiogram to assess any damage to the heart caused by COPD.
- Pulse oximetry to measure the degree to which the arterial blood is saturated with oxygen.
- A sputum test to check for signs of infection.

(NICE 2004.)

Additional complications of COPD

Cor pulmonale

Cor pulmonale is right-sided heart failure, which can develop as a result of pulmonary disease. Peripheral oedema is a common symptom. Cor pulmonale will usually require long-term oxygen therapy (LTOT) and medications such as diuretics to reduce fluid retention.

Anxiety or depression

It is important to be aware of the increased likelihood of anxiety or depression, which is more common in people with long-term illness. The current recommendations for treating anxiety and depression include the provision of support and medical therapy (NICE 2004). People may also benefit from stress management, relaxation techniques and support groups such as Breathe Easy Groups. These local groups are part of the British Lung Foundation and provide support for everyone affected by lung disease, including friends and family.

Treatment

COPD cannot be cured; however, with effective treatments quality of life can be improved. The aim of treatment is to reduce risk factors, manage stable COPD, manage exacerbations, optimise function and improve quality of life. Treatment usually includes smoking cessation, inhaled and oral medications, supplementary oxygen and pulmonary rehabilitation.

Smoking cessation

One of the most important aspects of COPD management is to stop smoking. Depending on the patient's readiness to change, he or she should be offered nicotine replacement therapy (unless contraindicated) and given access to support. Exercise professionals often see clients on a regular basis and are well placed to provide advice, support and encouragement.

Pulmonary rehabilitation

Pulmonary rehabilitation is a multidisciplinary programme of care, tailored to meet the needs of the individual. Comprehensive pulmonary rehabilitation usually consists of key components: exercise, education and psychosocial and behavioural interventions. It is usually offered to people with moderate or severe COPD; however, anyone who considers him- or herself functionally disabled (MRC 3 and above) should be offered pulmonary rehabilitation (NICE 2004). The goals of pulmonary rehabilitation include:

- reduction in symptoms;
- increased participation in physical and social activities;
- improved overall quality of life.

(ATS 1999.)

Medications

Oral and inhaled medications play an important role in the management of COPD and include drugs to control or reduce symptoms and improve exercise capacity (see table 11.6). The main role of medications in COPD is to relax and dilate the airways (bronchodilators), reduce inflammation (anti-inflammatory drugs such as steroids) and reduce the thickness of sputum, making it easier to cough (mucolytic medicines). Antibiotics will be prescribed for chest infections. Many patients will be on a combination of drugs to increase benefits. There are various methods for the delivery of inhaled medication including inhalers, spacers and nebulisers; the type used will depend on the preference and physical and cognitive skills of the individual and compatibility with other delivery systems used. In more severe cases, where oxygen levels in the blood are low, supplementary oxygen may be required.

Oxygen

Oxygen may be prescribed if the lungs are not able to deliver sufficient oxygen to the body.

Some of the signs and symptoms include:

- swelling in legs;
- skin has a bluish tinge;
- an increase in the number of red blood cells (polycythaemia) which indicates chronic hypoxia;
- raised pressure in jugular vein; or
- oxygen level is below 92 per cent saturation.

A PaO_2 (partial pressure of oxygen in arterial blood) measurement will indicate the amount of oxygen being transferred from the lungs to the blood. Oxygen may be required in the short term or long term depending on oxygen levels. Oxygen may be used during an infection or exacerbation.

Lung surgery

Surgery may be appropriate for selected patients with COPD and procedures include:

- bullectomy, which involves removing a large bulla (pocket of air) from the lung;
- lung-volume reduction, which involves removing part of the damaged lung;
- lung transplant, which is usually carried out in the final stages of lung disease and involves replacing the diseased lung with a healthy one. The limited supply of donors means that many people are not able to benefit from this procedure.

Exercise recommendations

People at all stages of the disease can benefit from exercise training. Exercise training improves the exercise tolerance and functional capacity of people with COPD, although it has little impact on lung function measurements or disease outcome (for example survival rates). The main benefits of exercise are improvements in exercise tolerance and symptoms of dypsnoea and fatigue (GOLD 2005). Exercise improves quality of life and additional benefits include:

- reduction in fear and anxiety;
- reduction of depression;
- improvement in efficiency of skeletal muscles;
- ability to return to work or continue employment;
- improved ability to carry out everyday activities.

Exercise intolerance People with COPD find it difficult to exercise due to dyspnoea and muscle fatigue and it is important to be aware of the factors affecting exercise intolerance. Exercise intolerance in people with COPD is mainly affected by ventilatory limitations, skeletal muscle dysfunction and cardiovascular and psychological factors.

Ventilatory limitation In COPD the loss of elastic recoil and airway obstruction increase expiratory resistance and make it difficult to expire normally. This expiratory resistance can triple the normal cost of breathing at rest (McArdle et al. 1991). The effects of increased airway obstruction and the reduced expiratory drive increase the time needed for expiration, which makes it difficult to adequately empty the lungs. This results in an elevated end-expiratory lung volume (EELV) and hyperinflation of the lungs. The diaphragm becomes shortened and flattened and less able to generate the force required for effective breathing. During exercise hyperinflation of the lungs increases (dynamic hyperinflation) contributing to dyspnoea and a reduced exercise tolerance (Berry and Woodard 2003).

Skeletal muscle dysfunction As well as lung damage, COPD also causes skeletal muscle dysfunction, characterised by a reduction in muscle mass and a change in muscle fibre type.

These changes may be caused by a number of factors, including:

- a decrease in levels of physical activity;
- hypoxemia (reduction of oxygen concentration in the arterial blood);
- chronic hypercapnia (high concentration of carbon dioxide in the blood);
- poor nutritional status.

(Berry and Woodward 2003.)

The combination of lung damage and skeletal muscle dysfunction contributes to the decrease in exercise tolerance that is characteristic of COPD.

Psychological factors Fear and anxiety play an important part in decreased exercise tolerance and the cycle of inactivity described earlier in the chapter.

Cardiovascular limitations Cardiovascular function is affected by an increased workload of the right ventricle caused by structural changes in the pulmonary circulation and dynamic hyperinflation (Sietsema 2001). However, people with COPD are more likely to be limited by other factors such as ventilatory limitations and skeletal muscle dysfunction.

Guidelines for exercise

There is no current consensus for the optimal exercise prescription for pulmonary patients; however, a comprehensive programme including cardiovascular and muscular strength and endurance training is generally recommended. The American College of Sports Medicine *Guidelines* (2005*a*) provides a framework, which can be adapted to meet the specific needs of individuals with pulmonary disease.

Cardiovascular training

Many patients with COPD reduce their levels of physical activity to avoid the discomfort of breathlessness. This results in a loss of muscle mass and a decrease in exercise tolerance, which usually results in a reduction in the ability to walk and carry out activities of everyday living.

Pulmonary rehabilitation usually focuses on a combination of strengthening and aerobic activities such as walking, stepping and stationary cycling. Stationary cycling is especially useful for people with COPD as the forward leaning position reduces the respiratory workload and the fixed arm position enables the accessory muscles to work more efficiently. This will enable clients to perform sufficient levels of cardiovascular training. Supported upper arm ergometry such as arm cranking can also be used within a cardiovascular programme; however, upper body cardiovascular exercise is less functional than leg exercise and at a given workload there is an increase in pulmonary ventilation, VO_2max and systolic blood pressure than at equivalent workload with leg exercise (ACSM 2001).

Until recently it was thought that people with COPD were unable to exercise at sufficient levels of intensity to elicit beneficial physiological adaptations, due to ventilatory limitations. However, recent research has demonstrated that patients with COPD may be able to achieve the aerobic training levels required for physiological adaptations (ATS 1999). Ideally, the intensity level of exercise will be based on the results of a sub-maximal exercise test such as a six-minute walk test (6MWT) or incremental shuttle walk test (ISWT), which are commonly used in pulmonary rehabilitation programmes (ATS 1999). If this information is not available a conservative exercise prescription is advisable, using exertion or dyspnoea scales to monitor intensity. The traditional method of monitoring exercise intensity using heart rate is less effective in people with COPD and an alternative approach using dyspnoea rating is recommended (ACSM 2005). A modified CR10 Borg scale is

often used to rate dypsnoea during physical activity (see box below). Patients are encouraged to exercise to a dyspnoea rating of 3–4 (moderate to somewhat severe). When determining exercise intensity, it is important to remember that high-intensity exercise may affect exercise compliance (Berry and Woodward 2003).

Modified CR10 scale

0	Nothing at all
0.5	Very, very slight
1	Very slight
2	Slight
3	Moderate
4	Somewhat severe
5	Severe
6	
7	Very severe
8	
9	Very, very severe (almost maximal)
10	Maximal

The amount of time that the patient can sustain exercise will depend on the health status of the individual and his/her level of conditioning. Most people with COPD find it difficult to maintain a higher intensity of exercise for prolonged periods and an interval approach to training is more manageable. This consists of short bouts of higher-intensity exercise (2–3 minutes) alternating with short intervals of rest. After an initial period of training the duration of each bout of higher-intensity activity can be gradually increased (ACSM 2005).

Muscle strength and endurance training

There has been limited research into the effectiveness of strength training in people with COPD. Peripheral muscle weakness contributes to exercise limitation and strength training is often used to supplement aerobic training within pulmonary rehabilitation.

Lower limb strengthening exercise

Exercises, such as sit to stand, squats, lunges and leg extensions are often included to strengthen the lower limbs, with an emphasis on the quadriceps muscles (which are commonly weaker in patients with COPD), the hip extensors and gastrocnemius. These muscles are important for everyday activities such as walking, getting on and off a bus and climbing stairs.

- Squats
- Sit to stand
- Lunges
- Seated leg extensions
- Leg press

Upper limb strengthening exercise

Current guidelines recommend that upper limb training is included in pulmonary rehabilitation; however, the research about upper limb training is less clear. Patients with COPD often develop compensatory mechanisms such as use of accessory muscles or fixing of the upper body to help with their breathing. They often have difficulty performing tasks that involve their arms as these compensatory mechanisms are removed. Activities that involve the upper limbs can provoke dyspnoea and fatigue. However, upper body muscular strength and endurance are required for activities of daily living such as shaving, brushing hair, etc., so it seems appropriate to strengthen the muscles of the upper body. The Australian Lung Foundation (2004) suggests focusing on strengthening the accessory muscle of inspiration (pectoralis major and minor, serratus anterior, latissimus dorsi and trapezius) and biceps and triceps for functional tasks. Exercises using body-weight, free weights,

resistance machines and therapy bands can be used to train the upper body.

- Chest press
- Wall press-up
- Lat pull-down
- Lateral raises
- Bicep curls
- Tricep extensions
- Seated row

It is important to focus on maintaining optimal posture, good technique and appropriate breathing during resistance training.

Respiratory muscle training

Respiratory muscle weakness may be a contributory factor to breathlessness, exercise limitation and an increased level of carbon dioxide (hypercapnia) in some people with COPD. Much of the research is focused on inspiratory muscle trainers using small hand-held devices. Muscle training with adequate loads does improve the strength of respiratory muscles in people with COPD; however, the benefits are not well established and more research is needed (ATS 1999).

Mobility and flexibility

Mobility exercise helps maintain the range of movement around joints. People with COPD often have a restricted range of movement in the spine, especially the thoracic spine. Mobility of the thoracic spine, including rotation, flexion and extension, is important for effective breathing. Spinal mobility can be included as part of the warm-up and cool-down. The exercises can be performed seated or standing, although seated spinal mobility is particularly effective for encouraging good technique. A combination of inactivity, ageing and breathlessness often leads to hunched posture and limited range of movement.

Stretching helps to maintain range of movement and can be used to address poor posture and increase flexibility. Consider a whole body approach with an emphasis on muscles that become shortened due to postural changes, for example the pectorals. Use appropriate positions and props such as therapy bands to ensure stability and effective technique. See table 11.4 for a summary of exercise recommendations for COPD.

Table 11.4	Summary of exercise guidelines for COPD		
Training guidelines	Cardiovascular	Muscle strength	Flexibility
Frequency	3–5 sessions per week. An individual with very limited functional capacity may require daily exercise.	2–3 (non-consecutive) days per week	3–7 days per week
Intensity	No consensus as to optimal intensity. 3–4 on Borg CR10 scale.	Begin at 50–60% 1RM and progress to 80% 1RM.	Lengthen muscle to point of tightness but not discomfort.
Time	20–30 min. (Interval training may be more appropriate for most individuals.)	1–3 sets of 8–10 reps	15–30 sec. Repeat stretches 2–4 times
Type	Walking, stepping, stationary cycling. Activities involving the upper body, such as rowing, may promote excessive dyspnoea in some individuals.	8–10 exercises using major muscle groups. Whole body approach with an emphasis on quadriceps, gluteals, hamstrings and gastrocnemius, accessory muscles of inspiration (pectorals, latissimus dorsi, serratus anterior, trapezius) and deltoids and triceps for functional tasks involving upper body.	Static stretch of all major muscle groups to improve joint range of movement and address postural changes e.g. pectoral muscles.
Functional	Include exercises that reflect activities of daily living such as reaching, stair climbing, sit to stand. Core muscle training, balance and coordination exercises address posture and balance.		

Adapted from ACSM (2005), Australian Lung Foundation (2004).

Key considerations

- Ensure appropriate screening to identify co-morbidities such as cardiovascular disease, osteoporosis and arthritis.
- Ensure medical management is optimised and client presents no exercise contraindications.
- Ensure ongoing assessment and modification of exercise programme in response to changes in health status.
- Progress exercise programme gradually.
- Late morning or early afternoon may be best time to exercise due to decreased dyspnoea.
- Avoid exercise in extremes of temperature and humidity (Cooper 2003).
- Encourage people to plan their exercise and activities to avoid doing too much in one day.
- Provide opportunities for development of social networks.
- Emphasise optimal posture and good technique.
- If client experiences excessive breathlessness, remain calm and encourage client to adopt a comfortable position and use breathing techniques learned within pulmonary rehabilitation. Leaning forwards, either seated or standing with arms supported, reduces the respiratory effort and will help relax the upper chest while encouraging the use of the lower chest during breathing.
- Provide support and encouragement to promote adherence.
- Living with a long-term condition such as COPD can be stressful. The relaxation component is an ideal time to practise relaxation techniques and effective breathing, emphasising the use of the diaphragm (see Chapter 7).
- Develop effective working relationship with local respiratory physiotherapists. This will enhance client care and provide opportunities for continued professional development.

Asthma

Asthma is a chronic inflammatory condition that affects the airways (bronchi) of the lungs. This causes narrowing of the airway, which is usually reversible, either spontaneously or with medication (Prodigy 2005a). However, in some people with chronic asthma, inflammation may lead to irreversible airflow obstruction (SIGN and BTS 2005). In asthma the airways are hypersensitive and constrict in response to a trigger, which results in a range of symptoms including shortness of breath, coughing, chest tightness and wheezing. Asthma can start at any age, but it more usually starts in childhood. Adult-onset asthma is usually triggered by exposure to substances in the workplace (occupational asthma) (Prodigy 2005a).

Cause

The cause of asthma is not completely understood; however, it usually occurs when the person comes into contact with a trigger that irritates the airways and causes the symptoms of asthma. Common triggers include:

- **Viral or bacterial infections** Infections such as colds, coughs and chest infections are common triggers. Some people with asthma may be advised to have a yearly flu injection; this will depend on their age and the severity of their asthma.

- **Exercise** For some people exercise is a trigger. Exercise is beneficial for overall health so it is important for people with asthma to remain as active as possible. Asthma symptoms that worsen during or after exercise may indicate poorly controlled asthma, and may require a review of treatment.

- **House dust mite** Some people are sensitive to house dust mites that live in soft furnishings, mattresses and carpets around the home.

- **Pollution** There is evidence that air pollution increases the likelihood of acute asthma attacks and aggravates chronic asthma (SIGN and BTS 2005). On hot days when ozone levels are high it is better to avoid exercising outside.
- **Animals** Pets such as cats and dogs can be a common trigger; finding a new home for the pet or excluding the pet from certain areas of the house such as the bedroom or living room might help.
- **Emotion** Feeling down or under pressure or trying to cope with ongoing stressful situations can trigger symptoms of asthma. A prolonged episode of laughter can also be a trigger.
- **Certain drugs** Beta-blockers, which are taken for heart disease and glaucoma, and non-steroidal anti-inflammatory tablets such as aspirin, can trigger symptoms of asthma.
- **Pollens and moulds** Asthma is often worse during the hay fever season.
- **Cigarette smoke** Smoking or being in smoky environments can irritate the lungs, trigger asthma and cause permanent damage to the airways.

(Adapted from Prodigy 2005*a*.)

Clients can reduce the severity of existing disease by avoiding known triggers. Sometimes a link is obvious, but sometimes there can be a delayed response to a trigger, making it more difficult to identify.

Some people may experience occupational asthma that is caused by exposure to specific substances at work, or they may already have asthma that is aggravated by substances or fumes in the workplace.

Prevalence

There are approximately 5.2 million people in the UK with asthma (Asthma UK 2005).

Approximately one in 10 children and one in 20 adults have asthma (Prodigy 2005*a*).

Signs and symptoms

These include:

- wheeze
- shortness of breath
- cough
- chest tightness.

People may have some or all of the symptoms of asthma including shortness of breath. The symptoms of asthma are often worse at night and are provoked by triggers such as pollen or exercise. Asthma does not always follow a predictable pattern and the severity and duration of symptoms may vary. During an exacerbation there will be wheeze and reduced lung function, which can be measured using a peak flow and spirometer (SIGN and BTS 2005).

Diagnosis

A doctor usually diagnoses asthma, based on typical signs and symptoms. Additional information will also contribute to a diagnosis of asthma:

- family history of asthma or atopic conditions such as eczema or allergic rhinitis;
- worsening of symptoms after using drugs such as aspirin, beta-blockers and non-steroidal anti-inflammatory medication;
- recognised triggers such as pollen, exercise, dust, or tobacco smoke.

Some of the symptoms of asthma are common to a range of diseases and conditions, which can make it difficult to diagnose. Asthma can also coexist with other conditions such as chronic obstructive pulmonary disease.

Objective measurements

Objective measurements such as peak expiratory flow (PEF) and forced expiratory volume in one second (FEV1) can be used in the diagnosis of asthma. In obstructive disease there will usually be a decrease in both these measurements; however, measurements may be normal if they are taken between episodes of bronchospasm. The following objective measurements demonstrate variability and reversibility of airway obstruction and can be used to confirm a diagnosis of asthma:

- more than 20 per cent daily variation on at least three days a week for two weeks, using a peak expiratory flow diary, is suggestive of asthma;
- more than 15 per cent (and 200 ml) increase in FEV1 after taking short-acting beta2 agonists or steroid tablets or an increase in airflow limitation after six minutes of running;
- more than 15 per cent decrease in FEV1 after six minutes of running.

(Prodigy 2005.)

Patients may be encouraged to monitor or home chart their peak flow readings as part of a personalised action plan. This can be used for the initial diagnosis and ongoing management of asthma (SIGN and BTS 2005).

Complications

If people do not have optimal control of their asthma, they will often feel tired and either underperform at work or need time off. In the UK approximately 1,500 people a year die from asthma (BTS 1997). Some people experience psychological problems associated with the development of the role of a sick person (Prodigy 2005*a*).

Treatment

General goals for working with people with asthma are:

- to maintain optimal control of asthma;
- to minimise symptoms during the day and the night;
- to avoid limitation of physical activity and work towards current recommendations for health;
- to maintain 'normal' lung function;
- to prevent exacerbations;
- to work in partnership with the client to encourage self-management of condition.

It is important to find a balance between optimal control and the inconvenience involved in taking medications and the side effects of medications (Prodigy 2005*a*). The client's goals need to be individualised and s/he needs to be actively involved in decisions about the treatment of his or her asthma.

Self-management

Self-management plays an important part in the management of long-term conditions. The Scottish Intercollegiate Guidelines Network (2005) recommends the use of a set of educational resources produced by the Asthma UK, 'Be in Control', which are designed to support self-management.

Avoidance of triggers

There is evidence that avoiding the exposure to a trigger or allergen may help to reduce the severity of existing asthma (SIGN and BTS 2005).

Smoking

Smoking cessation is advisable not only for general health, but it may also help reduce the severity of asthma. It is important that adults are aware of the health implications for children of passive smoking, which include an increased likelihood of developing respiratory disease and an increase in the severity of asthma.

Medications

Inhalers are the most common treatment to prevent the symptoms of asthma (for medications see table 11.6). Inhalers deliver the medication direct to the airways, minimising side effects. Inhalers are classified as 'relievers', 'preventers' and 'long-acting bronchodilators'. A stepwise approach is used to maintain optimal control of asthma. This involves stepping up treatment when required and stepping down treatment when the control of asthma is good. Any change the client makes to her or his treatment needs to be negotiated with the GP and written in her or his personal action plan.

Relievers (blue inhaler) Relievers are used to relieve the mild to moderate symptoms of asthma by dilating the airways. They are short-acting beta2-agonists and include salbutamol and terbutaline. If a reliever is required more than three times a week to ease symptoms, a preventer inhaler is usually prescribed.

Preventers (brown or maroon inhaler) A preventer is usually taken twice daily, once in the morning and once in the evening, to prevent symptoms developing. It does not have an immediate effect so it cannot be used for instant relief of asthma. Steroids are the drugs commonly used in preventers. Steroids are very effective in the management of asthma as they reduce inflammation of the airways. This causes a reduction of oedema and secretion of mucus into the airways, and decreases the likelihood of the airways narrowing.

Long-acting bronchodilator Salmeterol and formoterol are inhaled long-acting beta2-agonists, which may be prescribed in addition to the inhaled steroids if further control is required.

Corticosteroids Steroid tablets such as prednisolone may be required if the symptoms of asthma are severe or prolonged. If clients are on long-term steroid use (e.g. longer than three months) there is likely to be a reduction in bone density. A long-acting bisophonate should be prescribed to reduce the effects of steroids on bone density.

Exercise recommendations

People with asthma often have worsening symptoms when they exercise and this can be a barrier to increased levels of physical activity. This can lead to a cycle of inactivity with people avoiding activities that might make them breathless, resulting in decreased levels of activity and decreased fitness levels. Exercise contributes an increase in cardiopulmonary fitness and should be promoted as part of a general approach to improving lifestyle. Weight reduction is recommended for obese clients to improve asthma symptoms (SIGN and BTS 2005) and exercise can contribute to a weight-loss programme.

- Many people with asthma report that they feel better and have fewer symptoms when fit.
- Habitual physical activity increases physical fitness and reduces the likelihood of provoking exercise-induced asthma (EIA).
- Exercise training may reduce the perception of breathlessness through a number of mechanisms, including strengthening respiratory muscles.

(Ram et al. 2005.)

Exercise-induced asthma (EIA)

Exercise can lead to an increase in airway resistance in people with asthma, leading to EIA. It is important to give clients advice about how to reduce or prevent EIA by pre-treatment with appropriate medication and appropriate exercise recommendations (Ram et al. 2005). Exercise-induced asthma usually begins during exercise and symptoms worsen about 15 minutes afterwards (Asthma UK 2004). The mechanism behind EIA is not fully understood, but it may be connected to an increase in breathing rate, changes in airway temperature and airway drying.

Certain types of activity are likely to trigger exercise-induced asthma:

- exercising at higher levels (>75 per cent age-predicted maximum) of intensity is more likely to provoke asthma, although people with severe asthma may experience symptoms at lower levels of intensity;
- prolonged activity, such as long-distance running;
- exercise outside in cold, dry air;
- heavily chlorinated swimming pools.

(Asthma UK 2005.)

Exercise-induced asthma is usually related to poorly controlled asthma. Once asthma is more effectively controlled, the symptoms of EIA usually stop. If a client is on preventative treatment for asthma but still experiences problems with EIA, s/he may need to have a review of medication and an assessment of inhaler technique. Sometimes using an inhaled short-acting beta2-agonist is recommended just before exercise, to prevent the symptoms of EIA. This may need to be repeated during prolonged exercise (SIGN and BTS 2005). Asthma UK (2004) recommends an extended warm-up and cool-down to decrease the likelihood of EIA.

Exercise recommendations for people with asthma are in line with general ACSM (2005) guidelines. All components of the exercise programme and the basic principles of frequency, intensity, time and type will need to be tailored to meet the needs of the individual. See table 11.5 for a summary of exercise guidelines.

Exercise considerations and limitations

- Check that asthma is well-controlled:
  - Is sleep affected by night-time cough or wheeze?
  - Has asthma interfered with everyday activities or exercise?
  - Are peak flow readings lower than normal?
  - Is client using a reliever more frequently than usual?
    If the answer to any of the above questions is 'yes', postpone exercise. Advise client to go to his or her GP to discuss asthma control.
- Check that the client has regular check-ups with GP and has a written personal asthma plan.
- A dose of reliever just before exercise may help to prevent symptoms.
- Check client has appropriate medications such as reliever inhaler close to hand during exercise.
- Teach client to monitor exercise intensity using a rating of perceived exertion scale.
- A prolonged warm-up and cool-down will decrease the likelihood of asthma symptoms developing.
- Progress the programme gradually.
- Be aware of environmental triggers such as hot or humid days when ozone levels are high, or cold air. Use a scarf to cover the mouth and nose during cold weather.
- An interval approach to exercise, where periods of aerobic activity are interspersed with short breaks, is less likely to provoke EIA.
- Swimming is an ideal activity due to an environment of warm, humid air, and strengthening of the upper body.
- Make sure you know what to do in the event of an asthma attack. See Chapter 6, Health and Safety.

Table 11.5	Summary of exercise guidelines for asthma		
Training guidelines	Cardiovascular	Muscle strength	Flexibility
Frequency	3–5 days per week	2–3 days per week	Minimum 2–3 days per week. Ideally 5–7 days per week.
Intensity	55–75% HRmax 12–13 RPE	Stop 2–3 reps before fatigue (e.g. RPE 15–16)	To position of mild tension, not pain or discomfort.
Time	30 min (continuous or intermittent) activity	1 set of 8–15 reps	Develop or maintain range of motion for 15–30 sec and 2–4 reps
Type	Large muscle groups, dynamic activity	8–10 exercises, that train major muscle groups Target specific areas of weakness. Full range of movement.	Static stretch. Focus on muscles with a reduced range of movement.

ACSM (2005); Asthma UK (2004) .

Table 11.6	Medications for COPD and asthma		
Medication	Use/Action	Possible side effects	Relevance to exercise
Beta2-agonists Short-acting beta2-agonists Salbutamol Terbutaline	Quickly to reduce airway obstruction and symptoms of breathlessness and fatigue. Rapid-onset action and relief of symptoms for 4–6 hours.	Fine tremor in hands Nervous tension Headaches Palpitations Tachycardia Muscle cramps (rare)	Tachycardia May improve exercise capacity in clients limited by bronchospasm.
Long-acting beta2-agonists Salmeterol Formoterol (Oxis)	To control ongoing symptoms not relieved by short-acting bronchodilators. The duration of their action lasts up to 12 hours. They reduce bronchospasm and reduce hyperinflation.	As above	Salmeterol may help prevent exercise-induced asthma.

Table 11.6	Medications for COPD and asthma cont.		
Medication	Use/Action	Possible side effects	Relevance to exercise
Anticholerginics *Short-acting anticholerginics* Ipratropium	To relieve broncho-spasm. They reduce mucous secretion hyperinflation and increase FEV1. Can provide short relief for asthma.	Dry mouth Nausea Constipation Headache Tachycardia Atrial fibrillation	May improve exercise capacity in clients limited by bronchospasm.
Long-acting anticholerginics Tiotropium	Tiotropium lasts 12 hours. Maintenance treatment of COPD.		Tachycardia Atrial fibrillation
Methylxanthines Theophylline Aminophylline	Bronchodilator	Potential for toxicity and drug interactions. May cause tachycardia, arrhythmias, headache, palpitations, malaise.	May increase exercise capacity. Tachycardia and arrhythmias, palpitations.
Inhaled corticosteroids Budesonide, Fluticasone, Beclometasone	Reduce airway inflammation, oedema and secretions	Sore throat Sore tongue Hoarse voice Mouth infection (thrush) A prolonged high dose may lead to side effects for oral corticosteroids.	Consider exercise recommendations and limitations for osteoporosis.
Oral corticosteroids Prednisolone Methylprednisolone	Similar action to inhaled corticosteroids	Long-term use is associated with osteoporosis, weight gain, thin skin and bruising, altered diabetic control, weight gain, mood swings.	Consider exercise recommendations and limitations for osteoporosis. Altered diabetic control
Leukotriene receptor antagonists Zafirlukast Montelukast.	Blocks the effects of chemicals called leukotrienes that are produced in response of a trigger, in people with asthma		May be of benefit in exercise-induced asthma

Table 11.6	Medications for COPD and asthma cont.		
Medication	Use/Action	Possible side effects	Relevance to exercise
Cromoglicate	Mode of action not completely understood. May be of value in asthma with an allergic response.	Coughing, transient bronchospasm and throat irritation due to inhaled powder.	Can prevent EIA.

CARDIOVASCULAR DISEASE

12

This section will include the following:

- Introduction to cardiovascular disease (CVD)
- Angina
- Hypertension (high blood pressure)

Exercise as part of cardiac rehabilitation including post-myocardial infarction (MI), revascularisation procedures and cardiac surgery is not covered in this text. Please refer to Coats et al. (1995) and Thow (2006).

Cardiovascular disease (CVD) is an umbrella term that covers conditions that affect the heart and circulatory system, including coronary heart disease (angina, myocardial infarction), hypertension, heart failure, stroke and peripheral vascular disease. Cardiovascular disease is a leading cause of global death and accounts for approximately 17 million deaths a year (Smith et al. 2004).

The underlying cause of CVD is atherosclerosis. Atherosclerosis is a complex process, which involves the build-up of fatty streaks and atherosclerotic plaques in the walls of the arteries, in response to irritation or injury to the inner lining of the wall of the arteries. These plaques lead to narrowing of the arteries. Atherosclerosis can affect: the coronary arteries, causing coronary heart disease (CHD); the cerebrovascular arteries, leading to stroke or transient ischaemic attacks, or the peripheral arteries, causing peripheral arterial disease.

A number of CVD risk factors have been identified and include various genetic, environmental and lifestyle factors:

- advancing age
- family history of premature CVD
- ethnicity
- high blood pressure
- smoking
- elevated blood glucose or diabetes
- high cholesterol
- overweight/obesity
- physical inactivity
- unhealthy diet
- socio-economic and psychosocial stress.

(Smith et al. 2004.)

Multiple risk factors increase the possibility of an individual developing CVD; however, even single risk factors such as long-standing and severe high blood pressure can lead to premature CVD (Smith et al. 2004).

Current cardiovascular disease guidelines

With the development of new guidelines the focus of prevention has shifted from CHD alone to include CVD. The aim of CVD prevention in people at high risk is to reduce the risk of a cardiovascular event, improve quality of life and increase length of life. The new Joint British Societies (JBS) *Guidelines* (2005) recommend that CVD prevention in clinical practice focus on the following groups:

- people with established atherosclerosis including coronary heart disease, peripheral artery disease and ischaemic stroke;
- people with diabetes (Type 1 and Type 2);
- apparently healthy people who have a combination of risk factors that put them at high risk of developing symptoms of CVD (CVD risk of ≤20 per cent risk over 10 years).

All these people, whether symptomatic or asymptomatic, have some degree of athero-sclerosis caused by the same underlying disease process and they are considered high risk (JBS 2005). The Joint British Societies (2005) re-commend that all these high-risk people receive appropriate lifestyle and risk factor management interventions and drug therapies, with the aim of achieving optimal lifestyle and risk factor targets (See tables 12.1 and 12.2.)

Other people at high risk of CVD include people with single risk factors that are elevated, such as:

- high blood pressure ≥160 mmHg systolic or 100 mmHg diastolic or lower levels of blood pressure with target organ damage such as dia-betic retinopathy, stroke, transient ischaemic attack or peripheral arterial disease;
- ratio of total cholesterol to high-density lipo-protein (HDL), familial hypercholesterolaemia or hyperlipidaemia.

(JBS 2005.)

Cardiovascular risk assessment

The aim of cardiovascular risk assessment is to estimate the probability (percentage chance) of an individual developing CVD over a defined period of time. This is called total

CVD risk and is classified as low, moderate or high risk:

- high risk: total CVD risk of ≥20 per cent over 10 years;
- moderate risk: total CVD risk of ≥10 per cent–<20 per cent over 10 years;
- low risk: total CVD risk of <10 per cent over 10 years.

Cardiovascular risk assessment is used in primary care as a tool to guide practice and to help health professionals and patients make decisions about appropriate interventions, for instance in the areas of lifestyle and drug therapy. Cardio-vascular risk assessment should include factors such as ethnicity, smoking, family history of CVD, weight, waist circumference, age, blood pressure, total cholesterol and HDL cholesterol. The Joint British Societies Cardiac Risk Assessor Programme is recommended for use in the UK (NICE 2004c) and can be used to estimate the probability of an individual developing CVD over the next ten years. The risk prediction charts can be downloaded from www.bnf.org.

Cardioprotective drug therapies

All high-risk people will be prescribed an anti-platelet drug such as aspirin, and a statin to reduce cholesterol levels. People with established cardiovascular disease such as CHD may also be prescribed additional drugs including beta-blockers, ACE inhibitors and calcium channel blockers. See table 12.7.

Stable angina

A British Association of Cardiac Rehabilitation (BACR) Phase 4 qualification is the baseline qualification for working with CHD clients in the UK.

Table 12.1	Lifestyle recommendations for prevention of CVD
Smoking	All people who smoke should be encouraged to stop and be offered appropriate support, including access to smoking cessation specialists and nicotine replacement therapy (NRT).
Dietary management	Reduce saturated fats and trans-fats and replace with unsaturated fats such as rape seed oil or olive oil. Increase level of fruit and vegetables (a minimum of five portions of fruit and vegetables a day). Eat at least two portions of oily fish, or other sources of omega fatty acids, a week. Reduce salt intake to <6 g of sodium chloride or < 2.4 g sodium per day.
Weight control	Encourage people to aim for a body mass index (BMI) of 20–25. If this is too difficult for people, encourage more realistic target of 5–10 kg weight loss. Avoid central obesity.
Alcohol	Encourage people to limit alcohol consumption. For men limit intake to <21 (no more than 3 units in one day). For women limit intake to <14 (no more than 2 units in one day).
Exercise	Encourage adults to do at least 30 minutes moderate aerobic activity most days of the week. Exercise recommendations need to take account of specific conditions such as diabetes or obesity (see relevant chapters).

JBS (2005); Patient UK (2005).
*Adults with hyperlipidaemia are encouraged to exercise at least five times a week at a moderate intensity for up to 60 minutes. The aim is to increase calorie expenditure by exercising for 200–300 minutes per week, >2,000 calories per week (ACSM 2005).

Definition

Angina is a symptom, not a disease. Angina pectoralis describes the classic symptoms of chest pain, which is often described as a crushing pain, pressing or tightness. Stable angina has an established pattern; it is characterised by symptoms at a predictable level of exertion and it is well controlled with medication.

- CHD is the most common cause of premature death in the UK.
- Over 1.2 million people in the UK are diagnosed with angina.
- More men than women have angina and it is more common with increasing age.

(Prodigy 2003.)

Prevalence

- CHD is the most common cause of death in the UK.

Cause

Coronary heart disease (CHD) is the main cause of angina. CHD refers to the narrowing

Table 12.2	Risk factor targets for CVD prevention in high-risk people		
Risk factor	*People with atherosclerotic cardiovascular disease*	*Asymptomatic people at a high risk (CVD risk ≥20 per cent over 10 years*	*People with diabetes*
Body weight distribution	White Caucasian: men <102 cm, women <88 cm Asian: men <90 cm, women <80cm Body mass index (BMI) <25		
Blood pressure	<130 mmHg systolic <80 mmHg diastolic	<140 mmHg systolic <85 mmHg diastolic	<130 mmHg systolic <80 mmHg diastolic
Cholesterol Total cholesterol Low density lipoproteins (LDL)	<4.0 mmol/l or a 25 per cent reduction <2.00 mmol/l or a 30 per cent reduction		
Glucose (fasting plasma glucose)	≤6.0 mmol/l	≤6.0 mmol/l	≤6.0 mmol/l HbA1c <6.5 per cent

Joint British Societies *Guidelines* (2005).

of the coronary arteries supplying the heart muscle. Atherosclerotic plaques can develop over many years, causing narrowing of one or more arteries and the reduction of blood flow through the coronary arteries. This usually presents as stable angina, unstable angina, myocardial infarction (heart attack) or sudden cardiac death. People with other manifestations of atherosclerosis such as stroke or peripheral arterial disease are likely to have CHD. Stable angina is caused by the temporary shortage of oxygen to the heart muscle, which is often the result of emotion or exertion.

Risk factors for CHD

Risk factors are measurable factors that predict the development of CHD. The main risk factors that are routinely assessed in clinical practice are often classified as modifiable and non-modifiable (see table 12.3). Non-modifiable risk factors cannot be changed, whereas modifiable risk factors are susceptible to change.

Non-modifiable risk factors

Family history Family history is defined as CVD in a male first-degree relative, aged <55 years or in a female first-degree relative, aged <65.

Ethnicity Some groups within a country are at a higher risk of developing CVD than others because of genetic or racial factors (Smith et al. 2004). For example, South Asians (Indians, Bangladeshis, Pakistanis and Sri Lankans) living in the UK have a higher than average premature death rate from CHD.

Table 12.3	Modifiable and non-modifiable risk factors for CHD	
Non-modifiable risk factors	Modifiable risk factors
Age Gender Family history Ethnic origin	Smoking Inactivity Obesity Excess alcohol Stress High cholesterol Hypertension Diabetes

Age and gender Age is a major risk factor; although increasing age does not cause CVD, there is more time for the development of atherosclerosis, which can lead to CVD events (Smith et al, 2004). Women tend to present with CHD about 7–10 years later than men; onset in women may be linked to falling levels of oestrogen around the menopause, which causes an increase in cholesterol levels (BHF 2003). CHD is often considered a man's disease, but this is not the case. In 2001, 54,491 women died of CHD compared to 66,400 men. One in six women die from CHD, and after the age of 75 more women than men die of CHD (BHF 2003*b*).

Modifiable risk factors

Smoking is one of the main modifiable risk factors for CHD. Smoking influences the formation of thrombus, plaque instability and arrhythmia. People who smoke are more likely to have ischaemic heart disease and have a higher risk of dying from it. The more cigarettes smoked, the greater the risk. South Asian men, who are already at a greater risk of CHD, continue to smoke more than the general population. 29 per cent of the general UK population smoke, compared to 42 per cent of Bangladeshi men (BHF 2005*d*).

High blood pressure (hypertension) Persistently raised blood pressure is a key risk factor for CVD and people with high blood pressure run a higher risk of having a stroke or a heart attack. A person will be diagnosed as having hypertension if their systolic blood pressure is higher than 140 mmHg or their diastolic blood pressure is higher than 90 mmHg (NICE 2004*c*).

High cholesterol Cholesterol is a fatty substance produced by the body. It plays a vital role in the functioning of cell walls. It is made up of high-density lipoproteins (HDLs) and low-density lipoproteins (LDLs), which are responsible for transporting cholesterol around the body. People with high levels of LDL are at a high risk of atherosclerosis, whereas high levels of HDL appear to have a protective effect. Other blood lipids such as triglycerides also have a role in the development of atherosclerosis: a high level of triglycerides increases the risk of CHD.

Familial hyperlipidaemia Approximately 1 in 500 people in the UK have an inherited condition called familial hyperlipidaemia or familial cholesterolaemia. Diagnosis requires:

- cholesterol >7.5 mmol/l, or
- low-density lipoproteins >4.9 mmol/l in adults, plus clinical signs of hyperlipidaemia such as tendon xanthomas. These appear as lumps on the tendons at the back of the ankles or on the tendons on the back of hands.

People with familial hyperlipidaemia have an increased risk of CHD and aggressive treatment is recommended with lipid-lowering therapy and dietary advice (Patient UK 2004).

Diabetes In people with diabetes, good glycaemic control is essential. This has a beneficial effect on cholesterol and decreases the risk of coronary heart disease. Men with Type 2 diabetes have a two- to fourfold greater annual risk of CHD. Women with Type 2 diabetes have a three- to fivefold annual risk of CHD (BHF 2005c).

Psychosocial well-being The British Heart Foundation (2005c) identifies a number of psychosocial factors that are associated with an increased risk of CHD including:

- lack of social networks;
- stress related to employment;
- depression;
- personality (hostile).

Stress can result in chemical changes in the body, which can increase heart rate, blood pressure and cholesterol levels. Psychosocial factors can also have an impact on health-related behaviours such as smoking, diet, physical activity and alcohol consumption.

Diet An atherogenic diet can contribute to CHD in many populations (Smith et al. 2004). In the UK fat intake, especially of saturated fats, is too high and daily salt intake is well above recommended levels. Consumption of fresh fruit and vegetables is low and in the UK only 13 per cent of men and 15 per cent of women eat the recommended five portions of fruit and vegetables a day. There are also marked socio-economic differences, with people on lower incomes eating fewer portions of fruit and vegetables than people on higher incomes (BHF 2005).

Overweight and obesity Excess weight is associated with Type 2 diabetes, raised blood pressure and raised cholesterol, which are all risk factors for CVD. Central obesity substantially increases these risks. See Chapter 9 for further information.

Excess alcohol Alcohol needs to be considered within the context of dietary advice, in particular when an individual is overweight and needs to restrict calorie intake. However, a small amount of alcohol can be beneficial to the heart, possibly by increasing HDL. The pattern of drinking is important, with binge drinking associated with an increased risk of fatal myocardial infarction and stroke (Prodigy 2003).

Sedentary lifestyle A physically active lifestyle decreases the risk of cardiovascular disease mortality, especially CHD mortality (DoH 2001a). Only 37 per cent of men and 24 per cent of women currently achieve the current recommendations for health (BHF 2005c).

Social inequality Social inequality is considered a risk factor for CHD. Premature death rate from CHD is 58 per cent higher for men who are manual workers than for non-manual workers (BHF 2005). Factors such as psychosocial stress, behavioural factors and access to healthcare may contribute to an increased risk in people who are from lower socio-economic groups (Smith et al. 2004).

Signs and symptoms

The most common symptom of angina is a pain across the front of the chest. This may feel like an ache or discomfort, which can radiate to the jaw, neck, arm, or abdomen and is often accompanied by shortness of breath. Some people describe it as feeling like a band of steel being tightened across the chest, or a crushing weight. Although the term 'pain' is often used to describe the symptoms of angina, it is not always perceived as pain and some people describe it as a troublesome ache. It is often related to exertion and is relieved by rest. It can also be triggered by other situations, including:

- vivid dreams;
- eating a heavy meal;

- being out in cold windy weather;
- emotional stress.

Many people find angina very distressing and get frightened. These feelings can cause other symptoms such as palpitations, sweating and feeling sick. Angina doesn't usually last longer than 10 minutes with rest, or is quickly relieved by taking GTN. Some people find it difficult to tell the difference between the symptoms of angina and other chest pain such as:

- musculoskeletal pain
- referred pain from the thoracic spine
- oesophageal disorders
- pulmonary disease.

Chest pain is more likely to be linked to coronary heart disease in someone with two or more CHD risk factors; however, someone with CHD may still experience non-cardiac chest pain (SIGN 2001*b*).

Unstable angina

Unstable angina is the term used to describe angina that has changed in some way and is less predictable than stable angina. One or more of the following defines unstable angina:

- newly diagnosed angina;
- established angina that is getting worse, for example angina that comes on with lower levels of exertion;
- frequent episodes of angina, not related to exertion;
- sudden onset of severe chest pain at rest.

(BHF 2005*b*.)

Unstable angina is associated with atherosclerotic plaque instability and there is an increased risk of a myocardial infarction. (Refer to Chapter 6, Health and Safety.)

Diagnosis

The diagnosis of angina is based on history-taking to establish a clear description of the symptoms, including precipitating factors such as climbing stairs or emotions such as anger, anxiety or excitement. A physical examination and a number of both non-invasive and invasive investigations will be carried out to confirm the diagnosis of angina, which is really a diagnosis of coronary heart disease. There is no need to estimate cardiovascular risk in someone with angina, as they are already considered high-risk. According the National Service Framework for coronary heart disease, all patients with angina or suspected angina should receive appropriate investigation (DoH 2000*a*) and this may include referral to a chest pain clinic. The main investigations include:

Blood test A blood test will usually be carried out to check out previously undiagnosed diabetes, underlying anaemia or thyroid problems, and establish cholesterol levels.

Resting electrocardiogram (ECG) A resting 12-lead ECG records the electrical activity of the heart and provides information about the heart rhythm, previous MI and myocardial ischaemia. However, the resting ECG is not a very sensitive test for the diagnosis of coronary artery disease and a normal ECG does not necessarily exclude the presence of coronary artery disease (SIGN 2001*b*).

Exercise stress test An exercise stress test involves recording an ECG during an exercise test. The information gathered from an exercise stress test such as exercise capacity, blood pressure response and ECG changes can be used to diagnose CHD and to risk-stratify patients. If an individual has co-morbidities such as arthritis, an alternative test called a radionuclide test may be more appropriate.

Coronary angiography An abnormal exercise stress test is usually followed by a coronary angiography, which is used to aid diagnosis and support decision making about the most appropriate treatment. A coronary angiography is an X-ray examination of the blood vessels. It involves inserting a fine hollow tube (catheter) into an artery via the groin or the forearm and guiding the catheter under X-ray control into the coronary arteries. A dye is injected into the coronary arteries and X-rays taken to reveal the site and severity of blockages.

Treatment of angina

The aim of angina management is to alleviate the symptoms of angina, to limit the development of atherosclerotic plaques and to reduce overall cardiac risk. Management of angina involves lifestyle modification and drug therapy. In poorly controlled angina or if patients are classified as high risk, revascularisation procedures may be considered.

Lifestyle recommendations Lifestyle measures focus on the modifiable risk factors of CHD such as smoking, poor diet, physical inactivity, stress and excess alcohol. See table 12.1 for lifestyle recommendations.

Goal-setting and pacing Some people with angina find that they overdo things when they are feeling well, which can lead to an increase in angina or feelings of exhaustion, meaning they have to rest. Goal-setting and pacing can help people manage their angina more effectively and avoid overdoing things by planning their weekly activities. By gradually stepping up their levels of activity over time, it is often possible to return to activities that had previously been abandoned.

Relaxation Sometimes the pain and worry of angina causes an increase in adrenaline, which

can trigger a vicious circle: more worry causing a further increase in adrenaline, which increases heart rate and blood pressure, placing more workload on the heart, resulting in more angina. Some people find that simple diaphragmatic breathing exercises and relaxation techniques can help them remain relaxed and calm and more in control of their angina. See Chapter 7.

Medical management (see table 12.7)

The main aims of drugs therapy for angina include:

- short-term control of angina symptoms;
- long-term prevention of angina symptoms;
- secondary prevention of CHD.

Short-term control of angina symptoms *Glyceryl trinitrate* (GTN) is used for the immediate relief of angina symptoms. It usually comes in the form of tablets or a spray. Nitrates improve the blood flow to the heart by dilating the coronary arteries. If the symptoms of angina continue after three doses of GTN over 15 minutes, you will need to call 999.

Long-term prevention of angina symptoms *Beta-blockers* are effective in the long-term prevention of angina symptoms as well as reducing cardiovascular mortality and morbidity (SIGN 2001*b*). It is important not to suddenly stop taking beta-blockers, as there is some evidence that sudden withdrawal may cause a worsening of angina. A gradual reduction is recommended (BNF 2005). *Calcium channel blockers* relax the coronary arteries and reduce the force of contraction of the heart, and *potassium-channel activators* and *nitrates* improve the blood flow to the heart through dilation of coronary arteries.

Secondary prevention of CHD

Other medications may be prescribed to help reduce CHD risk factors, including aspirin, which reduces the risk of a blood clot causing a heart attack. An alternative drug, clopidigrel, may also be prescribed in the event of an allergy to aspirin. *Statins* may also be prescribed to lower the cholesterol level. If there is evidence of a previous MI and left-ventricular dysfunction (damage to left ventricle), *ace inhibitors* may also be prescribed.

Revascularisation treatment If a person is assessed as high-risk and has poorly controlled angina they may be considered for revascularisation treatment. This involves procedures to improve the blood supply to the heart muscle by widening the blocked arteries or replacing blocked arteries with grafts. The main revascularisation treatments include:

- percutaneous coronary intervention (PCI). This includes an angioplasty with or without a stent;
- coronary artery bypass graft (CABG).

Angioplasty An angioplasty is carried out to widen a constricted or narrowed part of a coronary artery. A catheter or fine tube is inserted into a large artery in the groin or the arm and, under the control of X-ray, is guided to the lumen of the affected coronary vessel. A guide-wire is threaded through the catheter and down the coronary artery until it is accurately positioned. An angioplasty balloon is then threaded over the guide wire and the balloon is inflated with sufficient pressure to widen the lumen. A tiny metal cage called a stent is usually inserted at the angioplasty site to help prevent re-stenosis (re-narrowing) of the artery.

Coronary artery bypass graft (CABG) This is a major operation that involves using healthy blood vessels, harvested from other parts of the body, to bypass the narrowed arteries and ensure blood flow to the heart muscle. There may be up to five grafts, depending on the site of the disease.

Exercise recommendations and considerations

Exercise has an important role in the management of angina and all people with CHD should be encouraged to increase their aerobic exercise within the limits set by their disease state (SIGN 2001*b*). Exercise training improves the ability of the peripheral muscles to extract and utilise oxygen and increases the amount of work that can be carried out at a given rate pressure product (heart rate **x** systolic blood pressure). As a result, sub-maximal exercise and activities of daily living can be performed at a lower rate pressure product, reducing the oxygen consumption of the heart (MVO_2) and decreasing the symptoms of angina. The ACSM (2005*a*) recommend setting the upper heart rate (HR) for exercise at 10 beats below the ischaemic threshold. If you have the results of an exercise stress test (on medication) you can establish a safe training heart rate range. The ischaemic threshold may vary depending on the type of activity, for example upper body activity is more likely to precipitate angina due to increased peripheral resistance. It is important to ensure that clients understand the importance of working within an appropriate heart rate range to prevent the onset of angina during exercise. Tools such as heart-rate monitoring and ratings of perceived exertion (RPE) can help clients to self-monitor. Angina scales can be used to rate levels of angina; however, these are more commonly used within exercise testing. A rating of three on the angina scale (see box overleaf) would normally be too severe for someone to carry on their activities of daily living and is reason to terminate an exercise test (ACSM 2005). If a client experiences angina during a supervised exercise session, document the exercise activity (mode, workload) and associated signs or symptoms, such as light-headedness or fall in blood pressure (AACVPR 2004). Advise client to stop exercising and follow the procedures for managing angina. (Refer to Chapter 6, Health and Safety.) Light-intensity resistance training, using higher repetitions and lower resistance (Gitkin et al. 2003), and a general flexibility component will contribute to a balanced exercise programme.

The exercise programme should be tailored to the overall needs of the individual, taking into account age, co-morbidities, fitness level, current physical activity levels, skill level, confidence, preference, lifestyle and personal goals.

Angina scale

0	No angina
1	Mild, barely noticeable
2	Moderately bothersome
3	Severe, very uncomfortable
4	Most pain ever experienced

(AACVPR 2004.)

Guidelines for exercise

It is important to be aware of any changes in the pattern of an individual's angina. There is an increased likelihood of an MI when stable angina becomes less stable. Unstable angina is a contraindication for exercise and it is important for the individual to seek immediate medical attention.

- Risk-stratify client in line with BACR guidelines (BACR 2000).
- Exercise may not be appropriate for someone who experiences angina at low levels of exertion (i.e. below 3 METs).
- Exercising in cold weather and after a heavy meal is more likely to trigger angina.

- Ensure client is able to recognise symptoms of angina, and especially their own, individual symptoms of angina.
- Encourage client to identify activities that trigger angina and, if appropriate, modify activities.
- Check that your client carries a GTN spray and knows how to use it.
- Record any changes in angina symptoms and notify GP.
- Some clients will benefit from taking pre-exercise GTN. Advice clients to discuss this with their GPs.
- Include a prolonged warm-up and cool-down to reduce the likelihood of angina.
- Advise client to remain seated for a few moments after using GTN as there is a risk of hypotension. The client can resume exercise if the symptoms ease, but you need to encourage the client to do some gentle pulse-raising activity as a warm-up.
- Ischaemia can occur without symptoms of angina (silent ischaemia) and is more common in people with diabetes.
- Level 3 instructors who are specifically trained to work with CHD clients should supervise clients with CHD in line with *Exercise Protocols for the Management of CHD Patients* (BACR 2005).

Hypertension

Blood pressure is the pressure the blood exerts on the artery walls. The pressure increases when the heart contracts and decreases as the heart relaxes. Systolic blood pressure (SBP) is the pressure exerted during the contraction of the heart and diastolic blood pressure (DBP) is the pressure exerted when the heart relaxes. This pressure is recorded as systolic blood pressure over diastolic

Table 12.4	Summary of exercise guidelines, angina		
Training guidelines	Cardiovascular	Muscle strength	Flexibility
Frequency	At least 5 times a week	2–3 times a week	Minimum of 2–3, ideally 5–7, days a week
Intensity	Training heart rate (THR) should be set at 10–15 beats below the client's threshold for angina. RPE will be a useful tool to use alongside THR.	Light resistance: 40–50 per cent 1RM	Stretch to a position of mild tension without discomfort
Time	30 minutes. An intermittent approach may be more appropriate for this client group. This can be achieved by exercising more frequently for shorter periods of time, such as bouts of 5–10 min performed two or more times a day.	1 set of 8–12 reps	Hold stretches for 15–30 sec. 2–4 reps of each stretch.
Type	Aerobic-type activities such as walking and cycling. Upper body exercise is more likely to precipitate angina than lower body activities.	8–10 exercises including major muscle groups. Dynamic resistance.	Static stretches with a focus on muscle groups which have a reduced ROM.

ACSM (2005*a*); Gitkin et al. (2003*a*).

blood pressure and is measured in millimetres of mercury (mmHg), for example 120/70 mmHg. Cardiac output and total peripheral resistance are the main determinants of blood pressure. Cardiac output is the total amount of blood ejected from the left ventricle in a minute and total peripheral resistance (TPR) is the resistance to blood flow offered by the peripheral vessels. This is influenced by the tension in the walls of the peripheral blood vessels and degree of vasodilation (increase in diameter) or vasocontriction (decrease in the diameter).

Blood pressure is expressed by the equation:

Blood pressure = cardiac output × TPR

The British Hypertension Society (2004) has classified levels of blood pressure (see table 12.5). A diagnosis of hypertension will be made if blood pressure is consistently >140/90 mmHg.

When there is no clear cause of hypertension it is called essential hypertension. Essential hypertension is the most common type of hypertension and may be linked to genetics and a number of lifestyle factors such as obesity or smoking. If hypertension is the result of an underlying definite cause such as kidney disorders or thyroid problems, it is called secondary hypertension. This section will focus on the management of essential hypertension.

Table 12.5	Classification of blood pressure levels of the British Hypertension Society (2004)	
Category	Systolic blood pressure (mmHg)	Diastolic blood pressure (mmHg)
Blood pressure		
Optimal	<120	<80
Normal	<130	<85
High normal	130–139	85–89
Hypertension		
Grade 1 (mild)	140–159	90–99
Grade 2 (moderate)	160–179	100–109
Grade 3 (severe)	≥180	≥110
Isolated systolic hypertension		
Grade 1	140–159	<90
Grade 2	≥160	<90

If diastolic and systolic measurements fall into different categories, the higher value is used to classify blood pressure (BHS 2004).

Prevalence

- Approximately 16 million people in the UK are known to have hypertension.
- It is more common in older people, with six out of 10 people in their 60s having high blood pressure (BHF 2005*a*).
- People of African Caribbean origin have a higher risk of high blood pressure than the rest of the UK population, which increases their risk of stroke.
- South Asian people living in the UK are at a higher risk from diabetes and CHD, so blood pressure needs to be carefully monitored.
- There is concern about under-diagnosis, under-treatment and poor blood pressure control in the UK (BHS 2004).
- Approximately 78 per cent of men and 66 per cent of women with raised blood pressures are not receiving treatment in the UK.
- Nearly 60 per cent of people currently being treated for hypertension are still hypertensive (BHF 2005*c*).

Cause

The exact cause of essential hypertension is unclear; however, it is likely that genetic factors predispose an individual to high blood pressure, especially when combined with environmental and lifestyle factors. The factors that contribute to hypertension overlap with the risk factors for coronary heart disease (Refer to Table 12.3).

Signs and symptoms

Most people with hypertension feel well and are symptom-free. If someone has really high blood pressure they may get headaches, but this is unusual. Other possible symptoms include sight problems, nosebleeds and shortness of breath (BHF 2005).

Diagnosis

A diagnosis of hypertension is made when an individual has a sustained blood pressure of >140 mmHg/90 mmHg (NICE 2004c). The Joint British Societies *Guidelines* (2005) recommend that all adults over the age of 40 should have their blood pressure measured within primary care as part of opportunistic risk assessment for CVD. Blood pressure can be affected by a number of factors including time of day, caffeine consumption and stress levels, so it important for blood pressure to be monitored on two or more occasions over a few months before a diagnosis is made. This process depends on the individual circumstances and someone with very high blood pressure may be reviewed more frequently or referred to a specialist if there are additional signs and symptoms.

Blood pressure is usually measured using a mercury sphygmomanometer, which is considered the gold standard, but due to health and safety concerns over mercury in the environment other automated or semi-automated devices are also being used. However, some conditions such as atrial fibrillation make it difficult to measure blood pressure using these alternative devices, and a mercury sphygmomanometer is more accurate. All equipment used should be validated, well maintained and recalibrated on a regular basis (NICE 2004c). Health professionals must be adequately trained and competent in order to take accurate blood pressure measurements. For full details about blood pressure monitoring methods see www.bhsoc.org.

Some people become very anxious when having their blood pressure measured by a health professional, and experience 'white coat' hypertension. Ambulatory blood pressure monitoring (ABPM) or home monitoring devices may be useful in certain circumstances, but their routine use is not currently recommended (NICE 2004c).

Hypertension increases the risk of cardiovascular disease, so it is important for a health professional to assess a hypertensive individual's overall CVD risk and treat the hypertension within that context. If there is no established cardiovascular disease, a cardiovascular risk assessment tool can be used. A number of routine tests can help identify other conditions, such as diabetes, or evidence of any target organ damage including the heart and kidneys. These tests will also identify any secondary causes of hypertension such as kidney disease. The tests include:

- a urine test to check for protein or blood;
- a blood sample to assess plasma glucose, electrolytes, creatinine and cholesterol levels;
- an ECG (12-lead) to identify any ventricular hypertrophy (enlarged heart, affecting the left ventricle) or evidence of myocardial ischaemia (shortage of oxygen to the heart).

Complications

Hypertension is the second most important cause of death and disability in developed countries (BHF 2005c). Hypertension affects the structure and function of the blood vessels and, if it is not managed effectively over a period of time, it can lead to organ damage including:

- kidney failure
- retinopathy (damage to eyes)
- left-ventricular hypertrophy, heart failure
- myocardial infarction, angina
- stroke, transient ischaemic attacks

- peripheral arterial disease
- an accelerated rate of decline in cognitive function (JBS 2005).

The likelihood of complications is increased by a combination of factors, including:
- co-morbidities such as diabetes and obesity;
- lifestyle factors such as a high salt diet and lack of exercise;
- risk factors such as family history, gender and ethnicity.

(NICE 2004c.)

Treatment

The aim of treatment is:
- to reduce overall cardiovascular risk;
- to work in partnership with patients to manage hypertension effectively through appropriate drug therapy and lifestyle modification.

Blood pressure can be effectively managed through lifestyle change and drug therapy in line with guidelines developed by the British Hypertension Society (2004) and the National Institute of Clinical Excellence (2004c). These guidelines give thresholds for drug therapy and lifestyle advice, based on an individual's cardiovascular risk.

Lifestyle recommendations

People often feel well and are symptom-free when they have hypertension. This can make it difficult for them to make the appropriate lifestyle changes. It is important for patients to be well informed about the risks of hypertension and the treatment options so they can take an active role in decision making about their health. Health promotion resources such as leaflets and audiovisual materials can be used to support one-to-one

Summary of British Hypertension Society (2004) guidelines

- The recommended blood pressure target for most people is a systolic blood pressure ≤140 mmHg and a diastolic blood pressure ≤85 mmHg.
- For people with renal impairment, diabetes or established cardiovascular disease the target is <130/80 mmHg.
- Anti-hypertensive medication is recommended for people with sustained blood pressure ≥160/100 mmHg.
- People with systolic blood pressure 140–159 mmHg or diastolic blood pressure 90–99 mmHg or both should be offered drug treatment if any of the following are present:
  - Target organ damage
  - A complication of hypertension or diabetes
  - An estimated 10-year risk of CVD ≥20 per cent

work with clients, and some clients may benefit from joining patient organisations or local groups that provide the opportunity to share information and experience and gain support. Some individuals who make lifestyle changes that lower blood pressure and reduce overall cardiovascular risk may reduce the need for long-term drug therapy (NICE 2004c). The following lifestyle measures are recommended in addition to those outlined in table 12.1:
- cut down on caffeine-rich drinks such as cola, coffee and tea;
- relaxation therapies such as stress management, or yoga and cognitive therapy, can reduce blood pressure. These treatments are not normally available on the NHS.

(NICE 2004c.)

Medication (see table 12.7)

Medication has an important role in reducing high blood pressure and the risk of cardiovascular disease. There are several types of hypertensive drugs, including beta-blockers, diuretics, calcium channel blockers and ace inhibitors. Generally a combination of medications will be offered depending on a number of factors, including age, ethnicity, presence of co-morbidities and response to treatment. Ongoing review is important to monitor blood pressure and provide appropriate lifestyle support. If an individual has a low cardio-vascular risk and her or his blood pressure is under control, it may be possible to reduce or stop medication; however, s/he needs to discuss any changes with the GP (NICE 2004c). Other medications such as aspirin and statins are also recommended for primary and secondary prevention of cardiovascular disease. Statins are generally recommended for people with hyper-tension and cardiovascular disease irrespective of baseline cholesterol levels (BHS 2004). The medical management of hypertension is currently being reviewed in light of new research, which suggests that newer approaches to lowering blood pressure may be more effective at reducing the risk of a heart attack or a stroke (NICE 2005).

Exercise recommendations and considerations

Role of exercise

Regular physical activity is an important life-style factor in the prevention and management of hypertension. Regular aerobic activity has been shown to reduce blood pressure, but the exact processes are not entirely understood. Exercise has an effect on the mechanisms that control and regulate blood pressure and immediately afterwards people experience post-exercise hypotension, which can last for two hours in healthy people and up to 12 hours in people with hypertension. In the longer term, the role of physical activity in preventing obesity, reducing insulin resistance and increasing the capillary density of muscle may contribute to a reduction in blood pressure (DoH 2004a).

Blood pressure response to exercise

During cardiovascular exercise such as walking, swimming and cycling there is a linear increase in systolic BP with increasing exercise intensity. This is linked to the increase in cardiac output during exercise. The increase in systolic blood pressure will depend on the intensity of the exercise and the individual's resting blood pressure. Diastolic blood pressure does not nor-mally rise in response to exercise, which is due to the blood vessels in the active muscles dilating, enhancing blood flow and reducing total peripheral resistance (McArdle et al. 2001). A decrease in SBP is an abnormal response to exer-cise that might indicate an underlying condition and is considered a contraindication to exercise.

Community exercise programmes do not generally monitor exercising blood pressure and this information is usually only available from the results of an exercise stress test. If you measure exercising blood pressure you need to be experienced and competent at taking resting blood pressure using a manual sphygmomano-meter, as most automated monitors are not designed to measure exercising blood pressure. It is easier to measure someone's exercising blood pressure while s/he is on a stationary cycle as you can keep the arm supported and relatively still.

During activity involving the upper body there is a different blood pressure response to exercise. Upper body exercise results in a higher systolic and diastolic blood pressure response than the lower limbs at a given VO_2max. This is because arms have a smaller muscle mass than legs, resulting in less vasodilation, greater resistance to blood flow and less reduction in total peripheral resistance.

Guidelines for exercise

Although the optimal training prescription to lower blood pressure is unclear, the ACSM (2005) *Guidelines* for cardiovascular, strength and flexibility training for the general population can be adapted. Moderate-intensity cardiovascular training is recommended as the primary form of exercise training for people with high blood pressure. The ACSM (2005) recommends an intensity of 40–70 per cent of HRR (55–80 per cent HRmax), but in the absence of exercise stress testing and in a community setting it may be more appropriate to exercise at a lower intensity of 40–<60 per cent of HRR (55–69 per cent HRmax). A resistance component of moderate intensity, using higher repetitions and lower resistance, contributes to a balanced exercise programme. The exercise programme should be tailored to the overall needs of the individual, taking into account age, co-morbidities, fitness level, current physical activity levels, skill level, confidence, preference, lifestyle and personal goals.

Table 12.6	Summary of exercise guidelines for hypertension		
Training guidelines	*Cardiovascular*	*Muscle strength*	*Flexibility*
Frequency	5–7 days a week. Daily exercise may provide optimal benefits due to the acute reduction in BP that follows a bout of exercise.	2–3 times per week	Minimum of 2–3, ideally 5–7 days a week.
Intensity	Moderate level 40–60 per cent of HRR (55–69 per cent HRmax). RPE 12–13 (Borg 6–20).	Low resistance/high reps	Stretch to a position of mild tension without discomfort.
Time	Continuous or intermittent activity of ≥30 min. Intermittent bouts (minimum of 10 min) accumulated throughout the day recommended.	1 set of 8–15 reps	Hold stretches for 15–30 sec. 2–4 reps of each stretch.
Type	Using large muscle groups, e.g. walking, cycling, dancing.	8–10 exercises including major muscle groups. Dynamic resistance exercises. Maintain normal breathing pattern.	Static stretch. Whole body approach with emphasis on muscles with a reduced ROM.

Adapted from ACSM (2005).

Special considerations

- If a client has high blood pressure, ensure that s/he sees the GP and is on appropriate medication before beginning an exercise programme.
- Discourage high-intensity aerobic or resistance training.
- Clients taking medications such as beta-blockers and diuretics may have an impaired ability to regulate body temperature and need to be aware of the implications of exercising in hot and humid conditions.
- Clients taking medication such as alpha-blockers, calcium channel blockers or vasodilators will require an extended cool-down to avoid hypotension after exercise.
- Encourage appropriate breathing technique during resistance training to avoid the valsalva manoeuvre (forceful expiration against a closed glottis).
- Discourage isometric activity such as over-gripping of equipment to avoid the possibility of an excessive increase in blood pressure.
- Avoid high-intensity or sustained upper body exercise due to increased myocardial workload.

(Adapted from ACSM 2005.)

Contraindication

Do not exercise if:

- Resting blood pressure is >180/100 mmHg.
- A significant drop in blood pressure during exercise is a contraindication to exercise. If an individual feels light-headed or dizzy during exercise advise him or her to stop exercise and refer to GP. (See Chapter 6, table 6.3.)

Table 12.7	Medications for cardiovascular disease		
Drug	*Purpose/action*	*Side effect*	*Exercise implications*
Nitrates Glyceryl trinitrate (GTN) (tablets or spray) Isosorbide mononitrate	Relax and dilate the coronary arteries, increasing blood flow to myocardium. Can be taken for immediate relief of angina or prior to undertaking activities likely to precipitate angina Prevent angina in the long term but become less effective with prolonged use. To treat heart failure.	Can cause headache, flushing or dizziness. Postural hypotension. Nausea.	Postural hypotension. Care with transitions e.g. floor-based work to standing. If client uses GTN spray and wants to continue exercising, be aware of possible drop in blood pressure. Can increase exercise tolerance by preventing angina and increasing ischaemic threshold.

Table 12.7	Medications for cardiovascular disease cont.		
Drug	*Purpose/action*	*Side effect*	*Exercise implications*
Beta-blockers Atenolol Metoprolol Acebutolol Propranolol Bisoprolol* Carvedilol* Sotalol** Esmolol**	Beta-blockers block the action of the hormone adrenaline. Reduce workload on the heart, and the incidence of angina. Reduce recurrence rate of myocardial infarction. Reduces hypertension. Stable heart failure*. Beta-blockers** can also act as anti-arrhythmic drugs.	May slightly raise blood glucose levels in someone with diabetes. Cold extremeties. Sleep disturbances and nightmares. Can precipitate bronchospasm in people with asthma or chronic obstructive pulmonary disease.	Symptoms of hypoglycaemia may be altered/blunted. Heart rate response suppressed. Risk of postural hypotension with floor-based work. Use RPE alongside adjusted target heart rate. Improved exercise tolerance.
Calcium channel blockers Amlodipine Felodipine Isradipine Nifedipine Verapamil Diltiazem	Reduce contractility of the heart muscle. Angina. Hypertension. Arrhythmia.	Dizziness, facial flushing,. ankle oedema. Postural hypotension. Constipation (Verapamil).	Verapamil and diltiazem can cause bradycardia.
Anti-platelets	These drugs decrease the clotting ability of platelets and may inhibit the formation of a thrombus or clot.	Indigestion. Nausea. Vomiting. Can bring on an asthma attack. Gastric bleeding.	None known.
Aspirin	Aspirin is used in both primary and secondary prevention. It reduces the risk of MI, stroke or vascular deaths by 30 per cent. Aspirin is also used in atrial fibrillation, stable angina and intermittent claudication.		

Table 12.7	**Medications for cardiovascular disease cont.**		
Drug	*Purpose/action*	*Side effect*	*Exercise implications*
Anti-platelets cont. Clopidogrel	Clopidogrel is used for the prevention of ischaemic events. It is often used if aspirin is contraindicated, or there are side effects.	As for other anti-platelets	As for other anti-platelets
Alpha-blockers Doxazosin Indoramin Prazosin	Hypertension not lowered by other drugs.	Postural hypotension. Urinary incontinence (women).	Postural hypotension. Care with floor-based work.
Anti-arrythmias Digoxin	To control arrhythmias. Supra-ventricular tachycardia. Atrial fibrillation. Heart failure (limited use).	Headache. Fatigue. Dizziness. Slow pulse.	
Amiodarone	Atrial fibrillation or flutter.	Photosensitivity. Metallic taste. Nightmares.	Possible reduced heart rate response. Possible reduced exercise capacity.
Flecainide	Ventricular tachycardia.	Dizziness. Visual disturbances.	
Anticoagulants Warfarin	Use in atrial fibrillation. for those at risk blood clots. Mechanical prosthetic valves.	Need regular blood tests. May cause bleeding or make it worse.	Check environment to reduce likelihood of tripping or knocking into equipment.
Angiotensin II receptor antagonists Candesartan Losartan Valsartan	Block the receptor site of angiotension II (a powerful vasoconstrictor).	Fatigue. Hypotension. Taste disturbance. Skin rash.	

Table 12.7	Medications for cardiovascular disease cont.		
Drug	Purpose/action	Side effect	Exercise implications
Ace inhibitors Captopril Cilazapril Enalapril Ramipril Lisinopril	Hypertension. Post-MI for LV function.	Dry cough. Rash. Renal impairment. Angio-oedema of lips and tongue.	There may be an increase in exercise capacity due to treatment of heart failure.
Diuretics **Group 1** Thiazide diuretics Bendrofluazide Chlorothiazide Cyclopenthiazide **Group 2** **Potassium sparing diuretics** Furosemide Bumetanide Spironolactone*	Hypertension. Heart failure*.	Diabetes. Gout. Hyperlipidaemia. Impotence. Hypokalaemia (loss of potassium).	Aching legs. Dehydration – encourage adequate fluid intake.
Group 3 **Loop diuretics** Lipid – regulating drugs	Reduce the progression of coronary atheros clerosis by decreasing concentration of low- density lipoproteins and increasing the high-density lipoproteins.		
Statins	Statins are used in both primary and secondary prevention of CHD. Statins reduce coronary events, all cardiovascular events, and total mortality. They are used in primary prevention	Gastrointestinal upset. Generally well tolerated.	Aching legs, otherwise no exercise considerations.

Table 12.7	Medications for cardiovascular disease cont.		
Drug	Purpose/action	Side effect	Exercise implications
Diuretics Group 3: Loop diuretics cont.	with patients who are at an increased risk of CHD. Statins are also used in secondary prevention of CHD, peripheral artery disease or a history of stroke.		
Fibrates Bezafibrate Ciprofibrate Fenofibrate Gemfibrozil	Reduce triglycerides and LDL cholesterol. Increase HDL cholestrol.	Gallstones. Rash. Gastrointestinal upset. Acute pain in calf or thigh muscle if kidney function impaired.	
Colestyramine (Questran)	Reduce LDL cholesterol.	Gastro-intestinal problems. Raised triglycerides.	

Adapted from BACR (2000), BNF (2005).

NEUROLOGICAL DISEASE

13

This chapter focuses on the following diseases:

- Multiple sclerosis
- Parkinson's disease
- Stroke.

Multiple sclerosis

Multiple sclerosis is a condition affecting the central nervous system (CNS). It is an auto-immune disease, which means that the immune system mistakenly attacks the body's own tissue. Nerve cells (neurons) carry messages around the CNS. A sheath of fatty tissue called myelin surrounds the axon, which is a specialised part of the neuron. The myelin protects and insulates the neuron and facilitates the smooth transmission of messages between the CNS and the organs of the body. In MS the immune system attacks the myelin tissue causing damage and inflammation (demyelination). This causes scar tissue (sclerosis) to develop over the affected areas, forming plaques or lesions. These lesions interrupt and distort the messages travelling along the nerve fibres. There is also evidence of damage to the axons, resulting in axon loss. These axons cannot regenerate and their impairment causes the progressive disability characteristic of MS. In MS these lesions can occur in multiple parts of the brain and spinal cord, causing a number of neurological symptoms. MS affects people in different ways, depending on the parts of the brain and spinal cord affected (MS Trust 2005).

Causes

The cause of MS is unknown. Current theories suggest an interaction between genetic and environmental factors. MS is not directly inherited; however, a combination of genes may make a person more susceptible to MS. The incidence of MS is greater as one moves further away from the equator (MS Trust 2005)

Prevalence

In the UK approximately 85,000 people have MS. MS predominantly affects young adults, with most people being diagnosed between the ages of 20 and 30. Women are twice as likely than men to develop MS (MS Trust 2004).

Signs and symptoms

The signs and symptoms of MS are varied and are not specific to MS. MS affects people in unpredictable ways; some people experience very few symptoms, some people experience different symptoms at different times.

Common symptoms include:

- Fatigue due to changes in the central nervous system can make physical and mental activity difficult. Depression, pain, and disturbed sleep are experienced. Poor diet, lack of physical activity and loss of fitness may contribute to feelings of overwhelming fatigue.
- Problems with balance and co-ordination; vertigo.
- Visual problems such as double vision (diplopia). The eyes might move from side to side or up and down. This is called nystagmus.
- Sensory problems such as numbness or tingling in the hands and feet.

- Muscle stiffness or rigidity (spasticity) and uncontrollable jerk (spasm). MS affects the control and regulation of normal muscle activity and maintenance of posture; this leads to uncoordinated movement, which can affect activities of daily living such as walking, getting washed and dressed, and leisure activities.
- Joint contracture due to tissues around the joint permanently tightening or contracting, which can occur if people have ongoing muscular problems such as weakness or spasticity that limits normal range of movement around a joint. This can lead to limited movement around a joint and in some cases pain.
- Pain: this can be neuropathic, caused by damage to the nerves in the brain or the spinal cord, or musculoskeletal pain (nociceptive). Nociceptive pain is often caused by lack of mobility and poor posture, or as a result of spasm and spasticity.
- Muscle weakness: damaged nerves, mainly in the spinal cord, affect the transmission of messages, causing muscle weakness. If these weak muscles are not used they atrophy, leading to secondary weakness.
- Shaking (tremor) and uncoordinated, clumsy movements (ataxia) can be very disabling, making it difficult for people to carry out activities of daily living, work and leisure.
- Anxiety, depression and mood swings;
- Cognitive problems affecting memory, concentration, speed of information processing, reasoning and judgement.
- Speech problems such as dysarthria, where weakness or lack of coordination in the muscles leads to slurred or slow speech and difficulty controlling intonation. People may also find it difficult to find words or form sentences (dysphasia).
- Swallowing problems (dysphagia) can happen when the nerves that control swallowing are affected.

- Bladder problems can involve difficulties with frequency, urgency, hesitancy and incontinence. This can be very disabling, making it more difficult for people to go out. Bladder problems are often combined with mobility problems, making it even more difficult to get to a toilet quickly.
- Bowel problems, including urgent need to empty bowels, constipation or pain.
- Changes to emotional state such as laughing or crying for no obvious reason.
- Sexual problems, which are caused by a number of factors including neurological, psychosexual and relational.
- Mobility (the ability to move freely). A wide range of factors can affect mobility including: fatigue, visual disturbance, posture, pain, depression, muscle weakness and spasticity. Inflammation around the spinal cord (transverse myelitis) can lead to leg weakness or paralysis.

(NICE 2003; MS Trust 2005.)

The most common presenting symptoms at the onset of disease include:

- A sudden reduction or loss of vision in one eye. This is called optic neuritis and is caused by inflammation of the optic nerve.
- Sensory problems such as pins and needles in the hands and feet.

MS is characterised by periods of remission followed by relapses (sudden episodes of symptoms). A relapse is thought to occur when a part of the central nervous system (CNS) becomes inflamed or damaged. The symptoms will depend on the part of the CNS affected. New or worsening symptoms may not necessarily be caused by a new episode of MS, but may be aggravated by a number of triggers such as infection, heat and humidity (MS Trust 2005).

Diagnosis

MS is a complex disease that is not easy to diagnose and there is no single test to confirm MS. The symptoms are not specific to MS and might be caused by other conditions. A neurologist will carry out a number of investigations to try to identify any changes in movement, reflexes and sensation that indicate damage to the nerve pathways. A number of tests may also be carried out to exclude an alternative diagnosis or to support the potential diagnosis (NICE 2003):

- A magnetic resonance imaging (MRI) scan of the brain and/or spinal cord can identify the site and severity of myelin damage.
- A visually evoked potential test monitors how the brain responds to patterns on a screen. The slower the response, the greater the myelin damage.
- A lumbar puncture obtains a sample of cerebrospinal fluid. This is analysed to check for the presence of antibodies, showing that the immune system has attacked the CNS.

Different types of MS are classified according to the patterns of progression:

Benign MS

In benign MS there are only a few relapses and little or no disability. If this pattern continues over a 15-year period the MS is classified as benign. See figure 13.1.

Relapsing/remitting MS

Relapsing/remitting MS is the most common type, affecting approximately two-thirds of people diagnosed with MS. At the onset many people have symptoms that come and go, with sudden relapses and remissions. A relapse typically occurs once or twice every two years and may last from 24 hours to a few months. During remission symptoms may disappear, but there may be some residual damage. See figure 13.2.

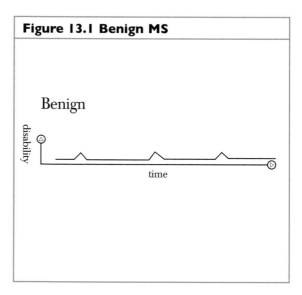

Figure 13.1 Benign MS

Secondary progressive MS

Approximately 50 per cent of people with relapsing/ remitting MS gradually develop secondary progressive MS. This usually develops during the initial ten years of the disease. There may be more or worsening symptoms and fewer remissions. See figure 13.3.

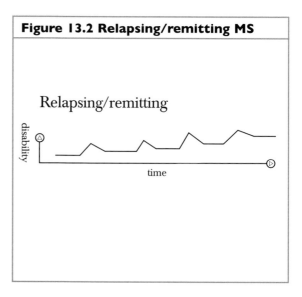

Figure 13.2 Relapsing/remitting MS

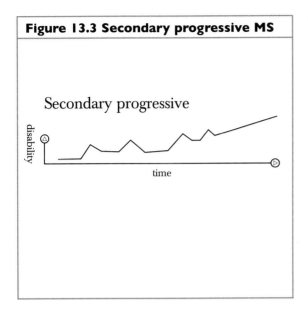

Figure 13.3 Secondary progressive MS

Secondary progressive

disability

time

Primary progressive MS

Approximately 10 per cent of those diagnosed have primary progressive MS. From the onset of MS the symptoms steadily develop and worsen, without relapses or remissions. See figure 13.4.

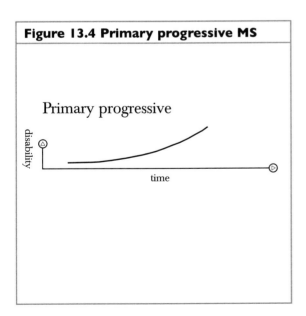

Figure 13.4 Primary progressive MS

Primary progressive

disability

time

Treatment

MS is an unpredictable disease, which can change from day to day or from one time of day to another. It is a lifelong disease that cannot be cured. However, it can be managed though a range of interventions. These include:

- access to a specialist multidisciplinary neurological team including physiotherapists, continence advisers, psychologist, speech therapists and occupational therapists;
- drug therapy;
- advice on maintaining a healthy lifestyle.

The National Service Framework (NSF) for long-term conditions recommends a person-centred approach with an emphasis on:

- provision of appropriate information and education;
- the opportunity for people to make decisions about their health;
- involvement in the development of a care plan.

(DoH 2005c.)

Medications

Drugs cannot cure MS, but they can be used to manage relapses, modify the disease and help manage symptoms.

Relapse management

Steroids are used to treat relapses. They help speed up the recovery from a relapse, but they cannot change the course of the disease. Steroids appear partly to suppress the immune system and reduce inflammation at the site of nerve damage. The NICE (2003) guidelines recommend the use of methyprednisolone in the short term (less than three weeks) and limiting the use to three times a year to avoid the long-term side effects of steroid treatment. The long-term side effects of steroids include bone cell degeneration, which can lead to osteoporosis.

Disease modification

Beta interferon 1a, beta interferon 1b and glatiramar acetate are called disease-modifying drugs. In the UK these drugs are licensed for the treatment of relapsing/remitting MS and secondary progressive MS, where relapses are a major feature (MS Trust 2005).

Other drugs used in MS

Some immunoregulators have proved effective in the treatment of other autoimmune diseases such as rheumatoid arthritis. This has led to the use of immunoregulators such as azathioprine, mitoxantrone, intravenous immunoglobulins (IVIg) and methotrexate to treat MS. Some studies show a reduction in relapse and a reduction in the progression of disability. However, these drugs are only used in specific circumstances (MS Trust 2005).

Medication to manage symptoms

Drug therapies are currently used to manage some of the symptoms of MS including bladder difficulties, depression, pain and spasticity, in conjunction with the support of a specialist neurological rehabilitation team.

- **Spasticity** Medications for spasticity generally act on the CNS and include baclofen, gabapentin, tizanidine and diazepam. These medications can cause drowsiness, muscle weakness, fatigue and dizziness and may have implications for exercise. Dantrolene is the only antispasmodic that works directly on the muscles, but is often not well tolerated. Cannabis is documented as improving spasticity and pain in people with MS, but it is not currently prescribed.
- **Bladder difficulties** Medications such as

anticholinergics and vasopressin may be prescribed to help with urinary problems.
- **Depression** Depression will usually be treated with a combination of drug therapy and psychotherapy. Medications such as selective serotonin re-uptake inhibitors (e.g. Prozac) can be beneficial for depression. Imipramine and amitriptyline may also be prescribed. These act on a variety of chemical neurotransmitters in the brain associated with mood regulation. Many of the medications prescribed for other symptoms of MS such as corticosteroids have depressed mood as a side effect (MS Trust 2005). Medication used for depression can cause an increase in postural instability.

Other therapies

Healthy eating

A healthy diet is important for general health and well-being. Linoleic acid may help maintain a healthy nervous system and is recommended for people with MS (MS Trust 2005). These essential fatty acids can be found in oils such as sunflower, soya and safflower and may help to slow the disabling effects of MS (NICE 2003).

Environment

People with MS are more sensitive to heat and humidity (thermo-sensitivity). An increase in body temperature may trigger a transient increase in symptoms (Karpatkin 2005).

Counselling

Counselling may help people develop coping strategies to deal with the change and uncertainty that are involved in living with MS.

Complementary therapies

There is limited evidence that some complementary therapies such as tai chi, reflexology, massage and neural therapy may benefit people with MS (NICE 2003).

Exercise recommendations

Appropriate exercise can help maximise muscular strength and endurance, flexibility and aerobic capacity. It can help:

- improve overall health and well-being;
- optimise and maintain function;
- reduce the disabling impact of relapses;
- reduce muscle wasting;
- reduce spasticity and avoid the development of contractures;
- improve posture.

(NICE 2003; MS Trust 2003.)

The exercise programme needs to take into account the client's health status, functional capacity, confidence, skills, preference and personal goals. A flexible, responsive approach is important to ensure the programme continues to meet the client's needs and reflects changing symptoms and energy levels. Exercise can contribute to fatigue, so it is important to plan exercise sessions to ensure an appropriate balance of rest and activity. Too much exercise may leave an individual feeling overtired and lacking the energy to carry out activities of daily living (ADL) and leisure pursuits. It is beneficial for the exercise professional to develop an effective relationship with the client's physiotherapist or healthcare team. This will facilitate communication and enable the exercise professional to respond appropriately to any changes in the client's health status and complement the work of the specialist healthcare team. See table 13.1 for a summary of exercise guidelines.

Cardiovascular

The type of activity will depend on the abilities and preferences of the client. Appropriate activities include cardiovascular machines such as stationary cycling, elliptical trainers, walking and water-based activity. Water-based exercise can help provide support for people with impaired balance and appropriate water temperature may help thermo-sensitivity (Karpatkin 2005). Intensity and duration may need to be adjusted on a daily basis according to symptoms and energy levels. The current recommendation of 30 minutes of moderate physical activity on at least five days a week may not be realistic for people with MS and will depend on the degree of physical impairment. The ACSM (2005) recommend a more realistic and achievable goal of 30 minutes of moderate physical activity on three days a week. This can be broken down into shorter sessions of 10 minutes and may be more appropriate for people with low levels of fitness, while ensuring sufficient energy and time to carry out ADL and leisure pursuits. A training heart rate of 60–75 per cent HRmax is generally recommended, but some individuals (older or more severely impaired) may need to begin exercising at lower levels of intensity (ACSM 2005).

Muscular strength and endurance

Muscle weakness is a common symptom of MS and everyday activities such as walking, climbing stairs and getting out of a chair become increasingly difficult. Strength training cannot alter the progression of the disease, but it can help maintain muscle mass and functional capacity. Lambert (2003) recommends training muscles unilaterally to accommodate differences in strength and range of movement between limbs. Fixed resistance machines provide more support and stability for controlled movement and may be more appropriate for people with balance and coordination problems. It is important to include activities such as small squats, step-ups and sit to stand, which can help an individual carry out activities of daily living and contribute to functional independence. It may be advisable for people with MS to perform strengthening and cardiovascular exercise on different days to avoid excessive fatigue. However, if an individual's condition is stable and their symptoms are mild, they may be able to tolerate aerobic training and strength training within the same exercise session. The ACSM (2005*b*) advise against strengthening work during an exacerbation, and suggest a focus on gentle ROM and stretching exercises if appropriate. Lambert (2003) recommends an exercise prescription for muscular strength and endurance for people with MS (table 13.1), but there is no consensus on the optimal prescription for resistance training. There are limited studies in this area and the variable nature of MS may make it difficult to develop protocols for strength training (Karpatkin 2005).

Flexibility

The muscle groups prone to tightness and contractures in MS are the hamstrings, gastrocnemius, iliopsoas and pectoralis major and minor (ACSM 2005*b*). Over time tightness in these muscles affects posture, balance, and gait and can have an impact on ability to perform activities of daily living. People with more severe MS may have contractures and they will need to be assessed for more specific treatments, which may involve long periods of stretching in plaster casts or removable splints (NICE 2003). For people with general tightness the ACSM (2005*b*) recommend performing stretching exercises once or twice a day, holding stretches for 30–60 seconds. Stretching programmes need to be tailored to meet the needs of the individual, taking into account ROM, balance and coordination.

Posture

Posture is important for efficient movement patterns, balance and respiratory function. In MS a number of factors such as muscle weakness, instability, fatigue and changes to eyesight can affect posture. Posture can also affect how an individual feels about her- or himself and how others perceive them. An exercise session is an ideal time to focus on standing and seated posture, with specific postural exercises and/or reinforcement of optimal posture throughout the programme. Betts (2004) recommends specific postural exercise for people with MS, with an emphasis on the position and the alignment of the pelvis.

Breathing

Breathing can become less efficient with changes in posture and a less active lifestyle. Breathing exercises such as diaphramatic breathing can play a role in improving posture, by exercising the diaphragm and abdominal muscles (Betts 2004).

Balance

Balance exercises are important for people with MS and can be incorporated within an exercise programme. Ensure a safe environment for people performing balance activities, with stable support such as a wall bar. If balance is a particular problem, a qualified Postural Stability Instructor (Falls Prevention) may be able to provide a more tailored exercise programme and appropriate level of support.

Exercise limitations and considerations

- **Fatigue** Be sensitive to daily variations in symptoms such as fatigue. This may be influenced by a number of factors such as medication, sleep patterns or temperature. Encourage exercise at times when energy levels are likely to be higher, usually in the morning.
- **Spasticity and spasm** Select a mode of exercise that is most appropriate for your client, for example some people experience

Table 13.1 Summary of exercise guidelines for multiple sclerosis			
Training guidelines	Cardiovascular	Muscle strength	Flexibility
Frequency	Structured exercise 3 days a week. ADL and leisure activities can be carried out on non-exercise days.	2–3 non-consecutive days a week.	5–7 days a week. Ideally twice a day.
Intensity	60–75 per cent HRmax. Use RPE to monitor intensity. Lower levels may be more appropriate for older or more severely impaired clients, until their fitness level increases.	40–80 per cent 1RM. Allow adequate rest between exercises.	To the point of mild tension but not pain.
Time	Build up to 30 min (continuous or intermittent). This can be broken down into shorter sessions e.g. 3 x 10 min.	1–3 sets 10–15 reps	30–60 sec. More prolonged stretching may be appropriate for people with contractures. Repeat each stretch 2–5 times.
Type	Low-impact, cycling, walking, treadmill, water aerobics or chair-based aerobics.	8–10 exercises. Focus on major muscle groups. Dynamic resistance. Relate to ADL. Modifications may be required to accommodate differences between limbs (strength and ROM).	Static stretching. Use props such as therapy bands or assistance by partner. Focus on muscle groups prone to contractures including hamstrings, gastrocnemius, iliopsoas and pectoralis major and minor.

Functional
Include activities such as small squats, sit to stand, stair climbing.
Include balance exercises to address postural instability.

ACSM (2005*b*); Lambert (2003).

ankle clonus (jumping feet), which makes foot stability during cycling difficult. Many people with MS have problems with one or all limbs going into spasms at different times. Betts (2004) describes a range of physical techniques involving posture and positioning that people can use to reduce the symptoms of spasm.

- **Relapse** Avoid exercising during a relapse. Gentle ROM and stretching exercises may be appropriate, depending on the severity of the symptoms. Exercise can be resumed when the person is in remission and the symptoms have either diminished or disappeared. The exercise programme may need to be reviewed following a relapse.
- **Balance, vertigo and dizziness** Use equipment such as stationary cycling as opposed to treadmill walking if balance is a problem. Ensure support is available for free-standing activities such as circuit training.
- **Muscle weakness** Muscle weakness can contribute to increased fatigue. It is important to exercise muscles to prevent atrophy. Gradually build up endurance and strength to avoid excessive fatigue.
- **Lack of coordination** Using fixed resistance machines can help provide support and stability and enable more controlled movement.
- **Sensory changes such as numbness** This may affect proprioception and balance during activities such as treadmill walking.
- **Thermo-sensitivity (heat intolerance)** Ensure the exercise environment is air-conditioned and a comfortable temperature. Encourage client to drink plenty of water before, during and after exercise to ensure adequate hydration. Some people may restrict their water intake to avoid problems with bladder urgency and incontinence. Dehydration might also contribute to fatigue. There is some evidence to suggest that cooling before or during exercise can enable a client to exercise for longer periods of time. Cooling methods include cold showers, ice packs and cold drinks.

- **Ataxia** Encourage use of handrail support in treadmill walking.
- **Cognitive loss, memory, attention, concentration** Provide step-by-step instructions and use visual and verbal cues to reinforce information.
- **Depression** Depression may affect adherence to programme. Consider a range of support strategies.
- **Visual disturbances** You may need to modify activity or use alternative equipment such as the handrail on a treadmill, or changing to a stationary bike.
- **Bladder and bowel problems** Ensure accessible toilet facilities.
- **Autonomic nervous system dysfunction** There may be an abnormal cardiovascular response to exercise in some people with MS. This has been observed in response to isometric exercise and incremental dynamic exercise.
- **Medications** Medications for MS may cause weakness, drowsiness, dizziness, postural instability and impact on cognition.

(ACSM 2005*b*; Lambert 2003; MS Trust.)

Stroke

A stroke or brain attack occurs as a result of disruption of blood flow to the brain. A stroke is also called a cerebrovascular accident (CVA). This is commonly caused by an occlusion, which leads to a lack of oxygen reaching the brain cells, or a haemorrhage (bleed) in and around the brain. Brain cells are damaged or die, affecting the function of the central nervous system. The brain cells around the damaged areas may recover as the swelling caused by the stroke goes down.

A transient ischaemic attack (TIA) is similar to a stroke and is often called a 'mini-stroke'. It is caused by a temporary lack of oxygen to the brain and can last from a few minutes up to 24 hours. The symptoms are the same as a stroke and indicate that part of the brain is not receiving enough blood. Unlike a stroke the symptoms soon go. It is important not to ignore a TIA, as people who have a TIA are at an increased risk of having a stroke. The greatest risk of a stroke is within the first 72 hours after a TIA (Royal College of Physicians 2004).

Prevalence

In England and Wales over 130,000 people have a stroke every year. Approximately one-third of people die within ten days of having a stroke, approximately one-third make a recovery and the remaining third are left disabled.

- Over 250,00 people are currently living with long-term disability as a result of a stroke.
- Nearly 60,000 people die from a stroke every year.
- Stroke has a greater disability impact than any other disease.

(Stroke Association 2005a.)

Causes

There are two types of strokes, ischaemic and haemorrhagic stroke.

Ischaemic stroke

Ischaemic stroke accounts for two-thirds of strokes. An ischaemic stroke is caused when the blood flow to the brain is reduced or blocked. The main cause of ischaemia is atherosclerosis, which leads to the narrowing of the arteries leading to the brain. This narrowing increases the likelihood of a blood clot blocking the blood supply to the brain. Within a few minutes of being deprived of oxygen the brain cells of the affected area become damaged or die.

There are different types of ischaemic strokes:

- A **cerebral thrombosis** occurs when a blood clot develops in the major arteries (carotid or vertebrobasilar) that supply the brain with blood.
- A **cerebral embolism** occurs when a clot develops in another part of the body (embolus) and travels to the brain.
- **Lacunar strokes** occur when there is occlusion in the small branches of the major intracranial arteries deep in the brain.

Haemorrghagic

Bleeding from a ruptured blood vessel causes a haemorrhagic stroke. This may be due to weakness in the wall of a blood vessel (an aneurysm) that ruptures. This can occur either in the brain (intra-cerebral) or in the arachnoid space between the skull and the brain (subarachnoid haemorrhagic).

Risk factors

The risk factors of ischaemic stroke overlap with the risk factors for coronary heart disease, and are often classified as modifiable and non-modifiable risk factors (see table 13.2)

The combined contraception pill (oestrogen and progesterone) and hormone replacement therapy (HRT) can increase the risk of stroke and the risks and benefits of hormone treatment should be discussed with a GP (Stroke Association 2006).

Primary prevention of stroke

Primary prevention of stroke involves addressing the modifiable risk factors for stroke (see

Table 13.2 Modifiable and non-modifiable risk factors	
Modifiable risk factors	*Non-modifiable risk factors*
• Hypertension • Smoking • Diet (high in salt, low in fruit and vegetables, low in potassium) • Excess alcohol • Overweight and obesity • Low levels of physical activity • High cholesterol • Diabetes	• Increasing age • Male gender • Asian, African, African-Caribbean • Positive family history of stroke

Stroke Association (2006), GP Notebook (2005*a*).

table 13.2) and managing existing medical conditions such as blood pressure, diabetes, atrial fibrillation (irregular heart rate) and high cholesterol. Stress and depression can contribute to long-term health problems and people should be advised to get help from a GP or health professional if this is a concern (Stroke Association 2006). Primary care plays an important role in identifying people who have multiple risk factors and a high risk of CVD. Risk factor prediction charts can be used to calculate the likelihood of a person having cardiovascular disease (including a stroke) within a ten-year period (BHS 2004). An asymptomatic individual with a CVD risk of ≥ 20 per cent over ten years is considered high-risk and should be offered the same advice on lifestyle and risk factor management as people who have already had a stroke or TIA (secondary prevention). See tables 12.1 and 12.2.

Signs and symptoms

The common initial symptoms of a stroke include:

• weakness;
• paralysis or numbness in one side of the body;
• drooping face or dribbling mouth;
• slurred speech, difficulty speaking or understanding speech;
• loss of vision in one or both eyes;
• confusion;
• headache;
• sudden problems with balance and coordination.

The most common symptom of a subarachnoid haemorrhage is a sudden, severe headache, which is often followed by loss of consciousness. Some people feel sick and have a stiff neck. These symptoms can be confused with a migraine or meningitis.

Diagnosis

The Stroke Association UK has expressed concern about the lack of awareness of the symptoms of a stroke in the general public and misdiagnosis of stroke by health professionals. It is important to recognise the symptoms of a stroke and act as quickly as possible to avoid delaying diagnosis and treatment. A stroke is a medical emergency and delay in diagnosis and treatment can lead to unnecessary disability and death. A tool called FAST has been developed to help people with accurate identification and is currently being used as part of a campaign called 'Stroke is a Medical Emergency' (Stroke Association, 2005*b*) to encourage people, including paramedics, to recognise the signs of a stroke and act promptly (see box below).

How to recognise the signs of a stroke (FAST)

Facial weakness
Can the person smile?
Has their mouth or eye drooped?
Arm weakness
Can the person raise both arms?
Speech problems/disturbance
Can the person speak clearly and understand what you say?
Test all three symptoms

(Stroke Association 2005*b*)

Diagnosis is based on the signs and symptoms of a stroke and the results of a brain scan to confirm the diagnosis. The Stroke Association (2005*b*) recommends that someone with a suspected stroke undergoes a brain scan and is given a diagnosis within three hours. A number of tests are commonly carried out to confirm the diagnosis and exclude other conditions

- CT scan (computed tomography) to confirm the diagnosis of a stroke and exclude the possibility of a bleed or other diseases;
- MRI scan (magnetic resonance imaging), which gives more detailed information than a CT scan, but is less effective at excluding other conditions;
- blood tests to check for diabetes, cholesterol and blood-clotting factors that may have contributed to the stroke;

- blood pressure measurements to identify hypertension;
- chest X-ray to identify any underlying conditions such as heart disease;
- ECG to identify abnormal heart rhythms;
- echocardiogram to check for underlying heart conditions;
- a Doppler or duplex ultrasound to check for narrowing of the carotid arteries.

Effects of a stroke

The effects of a stroke will depend on the age and health of the individual, the severity of the stroke and the area of the brain affected. A severe stroke can cause death, while a mild stroke can cause minor problems that might resolve over time. The left side of the brain is responsible for language and the right side of the brain is responsible for perceptual skills such as making sense of what you see, hear and touch, and spatial skills such as judging depth, size, distance or position in space (Stroke Association 2001). In most people the left side of the brain controls the right side of the body and vice versa. If the damage caused by a stroke affects the left side of the brain, there is likely to be paralysis on the right side of the body and problems with language.

Common problems

Cognitive problems

Mental processes involved in remembering, communication, attention, learning and perception (making sense of what you see and hear):

Memory Most people will have some problems with memory after a stroke. Some people have problems with verbal memory, which involves remembering language-related information such as names, while other people have problems with visual memory, which is non-language related and involves remembering faces and shapes. Losing prospective memory involves forgetting to carry out activities such as taking tablets. Total amnesia affects only a small number of people

Attention Problems with attention include:

- failure to concentrate on relevant or important information and filtering out less important information;
- difficulty focusing on important things such as the person talking to you or the traffic;
- being easily distracted.

(Moore 2001)

Communication Communication is one of the most common cognitive problems affecting people after a stroke. Language is usually affected when the left side of the brain is damaged; however, if the stroke has damaged the right side of the brain it can affect control of the muscles used in speech and affect concentration and the ability to organise language. The most common problems include:

- **Difficulty with language (dysphasia)**, which includes understanding what is being said (receptive dysphasia), making yourself understood (expressive dysphasia) and problems with reading and writing. Sometimes people feel that they are talking normally yet cannot be understood because they are missing out words or using words with related meanings.
- **Motor speech problems (dysarthria)**, which result from weakness or loss of control of the muscles used to make the sounds needed to speak. Some people have problems controlling their breath, using the voice to produce sounds and controlling the speed and intonation of speech. This can lead to slurred or jerky speech.
- **Difficulty in performing complex tasks (dyspraxia)** such as the control and coordination of movements required for

speech, can affect the person's ability to speak clearly and understand conversations.

(McLaughlin 2000.)

Perception Perception involves making sense of what is seen (visual perception), touched (tactile perception) and heard (auditory perception). A stroke can affect how people make sense of the world around them. Problems can include:

- inability to recognise objects and colour;
- difficulty judging space, distance or depth;
- difficulty understanding what is seen when it is looked at from an unusual angle;
- unilateral neglect, which means that people neglect one side of the body or the space around one side of the body. This may result in people bumping into things on one side of their body or forgetting to brush their hair on one side of their head.

Emotional and psychological problems

The type of problems experienced will depend on the site and severity of the stroke, for example damage to the right side of the brain may lead to impulsive behaviour, whereas damage to the left side of the brain is associated with anger and crying. Some of the emotional and psychological changes are related to physical damage to the brain and others may be related to the psychological effects of having to live with the consequences of a stroke. Common problems include:

- **Depression** Approximately 50 per cent of people who survive a stroke develop depression within the first year. Depression may be due to the disruption of electrical activity in the brain responsible for emotions, perceptions and thoughts; however, it is also linked to the effect of having a stroke and the impact of living with the changes.

- **Apathy** is common in people who have had a stroke. This may be linked to depression or be a result of damage to the area of the brain responsible for motivation and enthusiasm.
- **Emotionalism** refers to difficulty in controlling emotions, with exaggerated emotional responses and mood swings. Crying is a common problem after a stroke.

(Stroke Association 2005*e*)

Sensory impairment and pain

Pain and sensory impairment can be caused by a number of factors including:

- Immobility and existing conditions such as arthritis: musculoskeletal pain should be appropriately assessed and managed through exercise, improved seating, passive movement or analgesics (Patient UK 2005).
- Shoulder pain in the affected arm occurs in approximately 30 per cent of people following a stroke.
- Central post-stroke pain (CPSP) can cause large areas of pain in the leg and/or arm on the affected side of the body. CPSP may be caused by the brain's attempt to compensate for damage to the pain pathways and results in a loss of control over the mechanisms that regulate intensity of feeling. CSPS can be made worse by stress and emotional upset and some people find that relaxation, meditation, visualisation and gentle yoga may help (Stroke Association 2005*f*).
- CPSP may also respond to anticonvulsant medication or antidepressants (Patient UK 2005).

Paralysis, weakness and spasticity

Weakness on one side of the body (hemiparesis) and paralysis on one side of the body (hemiplegia) is a common problem. This is often accompanied by spasticity and muscle stiffness. After a stroke it is common for muscles to be floppy (flaccid) and weak. If the strength does not return, the muscle will begin to get stiff. It is important to encourage movement to avoid contractures (tightening of muscles, which makes it difficult to move the joint).

Treatment

Rehabilitation

The aim of stroke rehabilitation is to help people adapt to their impairments and enable them to participate as fully as possible in life. A range of assistance is available, including physiotherapy, speech and language therapy, psychologists, occupational therapy and specialist nurses and doctors. After a less severe stroke the undamaged area of the brain may take over and compensate for the loss of brain cells in the affected part of the brain. Recovery is fastest in the first three months following a stroke, but recovery may continue even after a year (Patient UK 2005).

Secondary prevention of stroke and TIA

People who have suffered a stroke are at an increased risk of a further stroke (30 per cent –40 per cent risk within five years). They are also at an increased risk of myocardial infarction or other vascular events. The risk of developing a stroke after a TIA can be as high as 20 per cent in the first month, with the greatest risk being within the first few days (Royal College of Physicians 2004). The Royal College of Physicians (2004) recommend that all patients should be given appropriate information on lifestyle factors including: smoking cessation, physical activity, diet and weight management, reducing salt intake and avoiding excess alcohol (see table 12.1). Haemorrhagic stroke is not usually caused by atherosclerosis; however, hypertension is a modifiable risk factor for haemorrhagic stroke so it benefits from medical treatment (Smith et al. 2004).

Medications

Drug therapy plays an important part in the secondary prevention of cardiovascular disease and includes medication for blood pressure, cholesterol and anti-thrombotic treatment (see table 12.7).

Blood pressure High blood pressure is a risk factor for stroke and it is important to manage it effectively. A target systolic blood pressure of <130 mmHG and a diastolic blood pressure of <80 mmHG is recommended by the British Hypertension Society (2004). Drugs commonly used to treat hypertension include diuretics, beta-blockers, calcium channel blockers, ACE inhibitors and angiotensin11 receptor antagonists.

High cholesterol Treatment with a statin (unless contraindicated) is recommended for patients with ischaemic stroke or TIA to achieve optimal targets (see table 12.7).

Anti-thrombotic treatment The Royal College of Physicians (2004) recommend that all patients with ischaemic stroke or TIA should be on antiplatelet drugs such as aspirin or clopidogrel or a combination of dipyridamole modified release and aspirin. Anticoagulants such as warfarin should be started in patients with atrial fibrillation unless contraindicated (e.g. in haemorrhage stroke).

Some medications such as baclofen, dantrolene and tizandine may also be prescribed for spasticity. The side effects of these drugs can include drowsiness, dizziness and fatigue.

Surgery A procedure called a carotid endarterectomy can be carried out to remove the fatty deposits from the carotid arteries to reduce the risk of a blood clot. Recent research indicates that carotid endarterectomy may halve the risk of a stroke in some people (Stroke Association 2005*g*).

After a subarachnoid haemorrage (SAH) surgery is carried out to seal off the aneurysm to prevent further bleeding (Stroke Association 2005*c*).

Exercise recommendations and considerations

After a stroke many people are deconditioned and are more predisposed to a sedentary lifestyle, which increases the likelihood of a further stroke or cardiovascular event. Physical deconditioning can limit functional capacity, affect the ability of individuals to carry out everyday activities and increase the risk of falls (Gordon et al. 2004). Exercise is beneficial for stroke survivors, but there are many barriers to physical activity (see box below), including physical impairments such as hemiplegia, spasticity and dysphasia, which are the primary neurological disorders caused by the stroke, and other factors such as intrinsic motivation,

Barriers to physical activity

- Degree of impairment e.g. hemiplegia and spasticity
- Access to appropriate (i.e. as to amount and type) rehabilitation
- Motivation and mood
- Depression
- Communication
- Cognition and learning ability
- Adaptability and coping skills
- Co-morbidities, e.g. cardiac disease
- Increased energy demands of physical activity leading to fatigue
- Impaired mobility and balance
- Perceived social stigma associated with physical and cognitive deficits
- Level of support
- Access to appropriate leisure facilities

(Adapted from Gordon et al. 2004.)

adaptability, coping skills, access to rehabilitation and appropriate exercise opportunities (Gordon et al. 2004).

These factors can make it increasingly difficult for people to remain active, and can lead to a downward spiral of activity leading to a decreased exercise tolerance, further deconditioning, muscle atrophy, osteoporosis and impaired circulation in the lower limbs (Gordon et al. 2004). Social withdrawal and social isolation is a major problem after a stroke and this can exacerbate depression, making it even more difficult for people to stay motivated and engaged in activity. Access to appropriate leisure facilities may help to address some of the external barriers to community-based exercise.

Exercise goals

- to improve overall health and well-being;
- to reduce the risk of recurrent stroke and cardiovascular events;
- to improve fitness levels, functional capacity and ability to carry out activities of daily living;
- to provide opportunities for the development of social networks;
- to encourage long-term behaviour change;
- to involve family and carers in the process.

It is important for the client to undergo a comprehensive pre-exercise assessment to identify neurological complications and medical conditions that require special considerations and an appropriate level of supervision. Many clients will have co-morbidities such as cardiac disease and it is recommended that stroke patients undergo an exercise stress test before starting an exercise programme (Gordon et al. 2004). This is not always realistic or practical and a lower-intensity exercise programme may be required to minimise the risks associated with exercise.

Cardiovascular

Although there is limited evidence about the role of cardiovascular training in stroke clients, a number of studies suggest that stroke subjects can improve their aerobic capacity and fitness levels following training (Brownlee and Durward 2005). Aerobic training may include leg, arm or combined leg and arm ergometry. In the absence of an exercise stress test it is important to have a conservative approach to exercise intensity and begin at very low levels of intensity, i.e. 50–60 per cent HRmax. A deconditioned client may need to exercise intermittently, gradually building up to a continuous aerobic bout of >20 minutes. Treadmill training is a functional activity important for everyday living and within the hospital setting treadmill walking is used for individuals with minimal motor impairments. An 'unweighting' device or harness can be used to lift the patients and decrease the amount of weight-bearing involved in walking. This increases safety and enables people who find it difficult to walk to get the training benefits associated with walking. These facilities are unlikely to be available in a community setting and treadmill walking may be inappropriate for clients with postural instability. Inclusive gym equipment can provide a more accessible and appropriate environment and enable clients with varying needs to exercise safely. Examples include:

- Straps on pedals or handgrips to help secure an affected lower limb: if straps are used to help secure an affected hand or foot, extra supervision may be required in the event of a fall as the client will not be able to extend an arm or leg to prevent a fall.
- Backrests and seat belts can be fitted to equipment to help with impaired sitting balance.
- Seated steppers are appropriate for people with poor balance and/or coordination. Some seated steppers have reciprocating levers that enable arm exercise.

- A stool or step can help people get on and off equipment such as an exercise bike. Encourage people to step up onto the step with the unaffected leg and step down with the affected leg.

(Adapted from Palmer-McLean and Harbst 2003.)

Strength

It is now accepted that strength exercises should be included in an exercise programme for clinically stable stroke clients. Strength training may contribute to an increased functional capacity and ability to carry out everyday activities and reduce postural instability. There are no current guidelines for how or when to initiate a resistance programme after an ischaemic or haemorrhagic stroke. The following guidelines are similar to those recommended for post-myocardial infarction:

- low intensity and high reps (12–15);
- 2–3 times a week;
- minimum of 1 set of exercises targeting the major muscle groups.

(Gordon et al. 2004).

Postural stability may be impaired and seated positions might need to be considered, or standing exercises using one hand to hold on to a stable support while exercises are done with the free arm.

Flexibility and neuromuscular

Flexibility training is important to increase range of movement of the affected side and prevent contractures. Many older people may already have orthopaedic conditions such as arthritis that may limit their ROM. Balance and coordination activities will be important to address postural instability and improve ability to carry out activities of daily living.

Table 13.3 summarises the exercise recommendations for stroke. The exercise programme should be individualised, taking into account the age, abilities, preferences, individual goals, skills and confidence of the client. It is important to be aware of any barriers to physical activity (see box on page 169) and find ways to provide a safe, effective and accessible exercise programme which meets the needs of the client.

Exercise limitations and considerations

- Behavioural factors may influence the selection of an appropriate exercise environment. For some people a busy, noisy gym might be too distracting, and encouraging the client to attend during quieter periods might help. A client who struggles with motivation and initiative might benefit from participating in a group circuit class, whereas someone who is prone to exaggerated emotional responses could benefit from one-to-one attention.
- Group exercise sessions with a high level of support may help address the issue of social isolation that people often experience after a stroke.
- People with perceptual problems might experience unilateral neglect. They may bump into equipment on one side of the body or forget to carry out exercises on both sides of the body.
- People might have difficulty in learning and remembering. Allow more time for teaching and reinforcing exercises. Try to encourage a simple exercise routine. Provide written instructions and label exercise machines clearly.
- Allow more time for communication. Make instructions short and clear. Sometimes it

Table 13.3	Summary of exercise recommendations for stroke		
Training guidelines	Cardiovascular	Muscle strength	Flexibility
Frequency	3–7 days per week	2–3 days per week	2–3 days per week
Intensity	50–80 per cent of HRmax; RPE 11–14 (6–20 scale)*	No consensus on optimal intensity. Low intensity, high reps.	Stretch to the point of tension, without pain
Time	20–60 min (continuous or intermittent, multiple 10-min bouts)	1–3 sets of 10–15 reps	Hold each stretch for 10–30 sec, 2–4 reps
Type	Large muscle group activities such as walking, cycling, combined arm–leg ergometry.	8–10 exercises including major muscle groups. Dynamic resistance exercises.	Static stretching. Aim to increase ROM on affected side and prevent contractures.

Neuromuscular
Coordination and balance activities 2–3 days per week (consider performing on the same day as strength activities)

*In the absence of an exercise stress test it is more appropriate to exercise at low to moderate levels of intensity (55–69 per cent HRmax). Compensate for lower levels of intensity by increasing the frequency and/or duration. Palmer-McLean and Harbst (2003); Gordon et al. (2004).

helps if the client repeats what you have told them in their own words. Some people might find it easier to understand the written word.

- Involve family members or carers in the exercise programme. They will be able to provide additional support, encourage home-based exercise and enhance exercise compliance.
- Be aware of the side effects of medications for spasticity such as drowsiness, dizziness and fatigue.
- Clients with altered body structure and function, such as hemiplegia, use much more energy walking than an able-bodied person walking at the same speed.
- After a TIA or stroke, ensure the client has been under the care of a medical specialist, is

on aspirin or equivalent (unless stroke was caused by a cerebral bleed) and is clinically stable. Liaise with GP and physiotherapist to ensure appropriate transition or return to community-based exercise programme.

- Many stroke patients will have co-morbidities such as cardiac disease, therefore it is important to focus on safety with appropriate screening, exercise programming, monitoring and client education.
- Monitor client's response to exercise and ensure clients are aware of warning signs and symptoms and what action to take, e.g. to stop exercise and inform instructor.
- Only work within your own levels of competence and confidence. Liaise with GP and physiotherapist and seek advice if needed.

- Where possible use inclusive equipment in line with Inclusive Fitness Initiative (2004).

(Adapted from Palmer-McLean and Harbst 2003; Gordon et al. 2004.)

Parkinson's disease

Parkinson's disease (PD) is a chronic, progressive, degenerative neurological disease that results from a reduction in the neurotransmitter (chemical messenger) dopamine. The reduction in dopamine occurs as a result of the death of dopamine-producing cells within a component of the basal ganglia (part of the brain) called the substantia nigra. The basal ganglia have an important role in the output of voluntary movement and postural adjustments (ACSM 2005). Over time more cells become damaged and levels of dopamine decrease, affecting movement, cognitive function, emotion and autonomic function. The symptoms of Parkinson's disease are also the main symptoms of a number of different conditions, which are grouped together under the umbrella term 'Parkinsonism'. 85 per cent of all people with Parkinsonism have Parkinson's disease. It is sometimes called idiopathic Parkinson's disease (IDP), which means that the cause of the disease is unknown. The remaining 15 per cent that have specific conditions that cause Parkinsonism, such as Alzheimer's disease or motor neurone disease or secondary causes such as viral infections, toxicity and head injury (Prodigy 2005g).

Causes

The causes have not yet been identified but are believed to be a combination of factors including:

- genetic susceptibility
- environmental factors such as toxins, e.g. pesticides.

Prevalence

In the UK approximately 120,000 individuals have PD. It is more common in people over the age of 50, and is more likely to affect men than women. PD can also occur in younger people, and is known as young-onset Parkinson's disease (Prodigy 2005g).

Signs and symptoms

Some of the main features of PD relate to movement, and include slowness, stiffness, difficulty in initiating movement and tremor. The symptoms of PD do not appear until there is less than 80 per cent of dopamine left in the brain, and these levels of dopamine continue to decrease over time. People are usually affected on one side of the body at the onset of the disease, but over time both sides of the body are affected. PD affects people in different ways and they may experience different combinations of the symptoms described.

Tremor usually begins on one side of the body, affecting the hands and arms. Over time it can spread to all four limbs. When the affected part of the body is supported and rested, the tremor will be more apparent. When the affected limb is moving, tremor is reduced. Tremor can worsen as a result of stress, anxiety or tiredness.

Bradykinesia (slowness of movement), **hypokinesia** (reduction in the amplitude or size of movement) and **akinesia** (difficulty in initiating movement) are the main features of PD. Common symptoms include feeling tired, difficulty in performing more than one motor task at a time or doing activities that involve fine motor skills such as writing or doing up buttons, and reduced speed and size of repeated movements such as walking.

Rigidity (muscular stiffness) is caused by an increase in muscle tone and resistance to passive stretch in both the agonist and the antagonist muscles around joints (ACSM 2005). This usually begins in one limb and over time spreads to the other limbs and other parts of the body. Sometimes the stiffness has a jerky quality and this is called *cogwheel rigidity*, and sometimes the rigidity has a slow, sustained quality and is called *lead-pipe rigidity*. When the trunk is affected, spinal rotation and extension become limited and postural reflexes are affected. It becomes increasingly difficult to perform functional activities that involve coordinating the trunk and extremities and limited trunk rotation makes everyday activities, such as turning over in bed, looking behind or getting out of a car, difficult.

Postural instability The impairment of postural reflexes affects postural stability, and when balance is challenged there is a delayed response and people are less able to right themselves and more likely to fall, often backwards. Over time their posture changes to a rounded upper back (kyphosis), a forward head position, and flexion at the hip and knee joints. People with PD may also find it difficult to shift their centre of gravity forward, and are at an increased risk of falling backwards when moving from sitting to standing.

Gait changes People may develop a characteristic gait with short, slow, shuffling steps, involuntary hurrying (festinating) and difficulty initiating movement. Gait is affected by the flexed posture, reduced trunk rotation and arm swing. Turning becomes more difficult and postural instability increases when turning.

Cognitive dysfunction Dementia, depression and hallucinations may also affect people with PD. Dementia and hallucinations may be part of the disease process, but they may be caused or aggravated by the medications taken for PD.

Autonomic dysfunction refers to the part of the peripheral nervous system that is responsible for the control of involuntary muscles. Features of autonomic dysfunction include:

- constipation and bladder problems;
- sweating;
- impotence;
- problems regulating temperature (thermo-regulation);
- problems with swallowing (dysphagia);
- in the later stages postural hypotension is common, although this may be aggravated by medications for PD.

Pulmonary Some people with PD may experience respiratory problems (obstructive and restrictive), which may be linked to changes in functioning of the respiratory muscles, loss of flexibility in the trunk and postural changes (ACSM 2005).

Other features of Parkinson's disease include:

- sleep disturbances;
- altered sense of smell;
- changes in speech;
- lack of facial expression.

The symptoms will generally get worse over time; however, the rate of progression will vary from person to person.

Diagnosis

Parkinson's disease is difficult to diagnose as many of the signs and symptoms may be due to other disorders or secondary causes such as:

- Alzheimer's disease
- motor neurone disease
- antipsychotic drugs
- cerebrovascular disease
- head injuries (e.g. in boxers)
- toxicity (e.g. carbon monoxide).

Patients with suspected PD should be referred to a neurologist or physician with a special interest in the disease for a diagnosis to be confirmed.

Treatment

There are no treatments to cure PD, or to prevent the progression of the disease. Current treatments aim to ease the symptoms. If someone has mild symptoms they will often decide to postpone drug therapy and focus on improving their lifestyle through healthy eating, exercise and relaxation. As the disease progresses and symptoms worsen, drug therapy will be introduced. Drug therapy and a healthy lifestyle (nutritious diet, relaxation and exercises) are essential components in the management of PD. Therapies such as physio-, occupational and speech therapy play an important part in the ongoing management of the disease.

Healthy eating

The current guidelines for healthy eating promoted by the British Nutrition Foundation (2005) are recommended for people with PD. Specific advice includes:

- Increasing intake of fluid and high-fibre foods and increasing physical activity levels are recommended for constipation.
- Timing of medications may need to be discussed with GP as protein in foods can interfere with the absorption of some medication such as Levodopa (Parkinson's Disease Society 2003*b*).
- People with chewing and swallowing problems may need specialist advice from a speech and language specialist.

Relaxation

When a person has PD a lot of concentration and mental energy is used to carry out relatively simple activities of daily living. Relaxation can have a positive impact on well-being and can be used in isolation or within an exercise programme. Complementary therapies such as massage therapy and reflexology and relaxation techniques may also help relieve symptoms and help people with stress and low moods (Parkinson's Disease Society 2005*a*).

Medication (table 13.4)

The main aim of drug treatment is to control symptoms and improve quality of life. The medication can control symptoms by:

- increasing the levels of dopamine in the brain;
- stimulating the parts of the brain where dopamine works;
- blocking the action of chemicals such as acetylcholine that affect dopamine;
- blocking the action of other enzymes that affect dopamine.

(Parkinson's Disease Society 2005*b*.)

There are complications associated with the long-term use of PD drug therapy, caused by an interaction between the disease and the drugs. People can experience 'early wearing-off', where the effect of the medication does not last as long as necessary and loses its effect before the next dose. 'On/off syndrome' can also occur, where symptoms such as dyskinesia (involuntary movements) start and stop unexpectedly (Parkinson's Disease Society 2004*b*). People with PD usually have postural instability and the drugs used to treat the symptoms can cause dizziness and postural hypotension. Depression is more common in people with PD and some people may be on antidepressants, which can have a sedative effect and cause sleepiness, which in turn has implications for exercise.

Table 13.4 Medication for Parkinson's disease

Name of medication	Action/purpose	Side effects	Implications for exercise
Dopaminergics Levodopa Madopar Sinemet	Levodopa is a chemical that the brain converts into dopamine. It can dramatically improve symptoms of PD.	Nausea and vomiting. Orthostatic hypotension. Cardiac arrhythmias. Excessive drowsiness, sudden onset of sleep. Motor complications over time such as dyskinesia (involuntary movements), freezing and motor fluctuations.	Othostatic (postural hypotension). Timing of exercise. Motor complications. Cardiac arrhythmias. Improvement in stiffness and slowness of movement. Longer-term motor fluctuations.
Dopamine agonists Bromocriptine Cabergoline Pergolide Pramipexole Ropinirole Apomorphine	Dopamine agonists stimulate the part of the brain where dopamine works. They are often used in addition to levodopa.	Nausea and vomiting. Confusion or hallucinations, drowsiness.	
Anticholergics Trihexyphenidyl Benztropine Orphenadrine Procyclidine	Blocks the action of the chemical messenger acetylcholine. Useful for younger people with mild symptoms. More effective at improving tremor than slowness and stiffness. Reduces production of saliva when drooling is problematic, and reduces bladder contractions (urge incontinence).	Cardiac irregularities, mood changes, memory loss, confusion, blurred vision, dry mouth, nausea and vomiting. Not used in the elderly due to the side effects, which might be mental confusion and heightened glaucoma.	Be aware of possible cardiac irregularities. Improvement in tremor more than slowness or stiffness.
Monoamine oxidase type B inhibitor Selegiline	Blocks the enzyme MAO-B that breaks down dopamine in the brain.	Insomnia, headaches, sweating	
COMT inhibitor Entacapone Tolcapone	Prolongs the action of levodopa by blocking the action of an enzyme that breaks it down. Reduces symptoms.	Nausea, vomiting and diarrhoea. Can exacerbate involuntary movement (dyskinesia).	Possible exacerbation of involuntary movement (dyskinesia).

BNF (2005); Parkinson's Disease Society (2005).

Exercise limitations and considerations

There is very limited research about the benefits of exercise in people with PD, but regular physical activity can influence survival rate by preventing the deconditioning and decline associated with inactivity (Northumbria University 2005). There is no current evidence to suggest that exercise can affect the progression of the disease; however, it can help:

- improve quality of life;
- increase fitness levels;
- improve balance, posture, mobility and gait;
- alleviate some of the symptoms of the disease, including stiffness and slowness of movement;
- promote independence.

For people with mild to moderate PD a general fitness programme following ACSM guidelines is probably appropriate (ACSM 2005*b*). The programme should be individualised and take into account the limitations of the client, including age and co-morbidities such as heart disease. It is important for the exercise professional to be in partnership with other health professionals working with the client, such as a physiotherapist who has more specialised skills, knowledge and experience of working with people with PD. This partnership becomes increasingly vital as the disease progresses and a more specialised programme addressing gait and balance is required. Orofacial and breathing techniques may also be included within a specialist programme. The progression of the disease will determine the level of supervision required and the exercise environment, which may need to change to meet the specific needs of the client. See table 13.5 for a summary of exercise guidelines.

Cardiovascular training

The evidence for cardiovascular exercise in people with PD is limited, but it may be appropriate to maintain aerobic capacity in people with mild or moderate levels. People with PD often have little physical activity, leading to low levels of cardiorespiratory fitness. Cardiovascular training is important for overall health and well-being as well as cardiovascular health. Where possible functional activities, such as walking, are recommended. Treadmill walking may not be a safe option, although this will depend on the individual's symptoms. If postural instability is a concern a stationary bike or upper body ergometer may be more appropriate. Equipment such as cross trainers, which involve the upper and lower body, are a good option as they encourage a good ROM and encourage trunk rotation.

Muscular strength and endurance

The ACSM (2005*b*) acknowledge the lack of research in this client group. They suggest using the ACSM guidelines for the general population, provided the programme takes into account age, co-morbidities, individual limitations and impairments.

Further considerations for this component include:

- Ensure client performs an adequate warm-up that includes low-level aerobic activity, joint mobility exercise and stretches before beginning a resistance programme.
- Reinforce good posture during muscle strength and endurance activities.
- Emphasise extensor muscles such as lower and middle trapezius, rhomboids, erector spinae, gluteus maximus and quadriceps.
- Include exercises such as standing squats, prone squeezes, leg extensions, calf raises, back extensions and toe lifts.

- Where possible use functional positions, e.g. standing squats.
- Use sound and visual cues such as clapping, body language or a metronome to help with movement and timing.

(Adapted from ACSM 2005.)

Flexibility

Low levels of physical activity and poor posture can lead to reduced ROM around joints and tight muscles. This can eventually lead to the development of contractures in certain muscle groups and a reduced ROM in hip and knee extension, dorsi-flexion, shoulder flexion, external shoulder rotation, trunk extension and axial rotation (ACSM 2005). There is limited research on the effectiveness of flexibility training for people with PD. A general stretching programme is appropriate for people with mild muscle tightness, but people with severe muscle tightness or muscle contractures will require a more specialised stretching programme delivered by a physiotherapist. Refer to Norris (2004) for comprehensive information on the principles and practice of stretching.

Further considerations for this component include:

- Tailor the stretch programme, taking into account individual ROM and stability.
- Consider appropriate positions, including floor, standing, seated and using a couch for people who find it difficult to get down onto the floor.
- Reinforce optimal posture.
- Use a range of tools such as therapy bands, exercise balls and foam rollers and touch to encourage ROM and enhance stretching.
- Include a range of stretches with an emphasis on gastrocnemius, soleus, hamstring, hip flexor and pectoral stretch. Spinal extension, lateral flexion and rotation are particularly important to increase ROM in the spine.

- Include stretching exercises for the hands.
- Encourage a daily stretching programme.

Posture

It is important to reinforce optimal posture throughout the exercise programme. Poor posture not only affects walking and postural stability, but also breathing, swallowing and speaking loudly and clearly. A stooped posture can also affect the way people feel about themselves and the way other people perceive them. The Parkinson Society for Canada (2003) emphasises the importance of checking seated and standing posture throughout the day and recommends a number of specific exercises to practise daily including:

- Lie on the floor with legs outstretched. Provide support under head to ensure spinal alignment. Allow gravity to gently stretch out and lengthen tightened muscles.
- Back extension from a prone lying position to strengthen the back extensors.
- Shoulder squeezes (seated or lying prone) to strengthen the shoulder retractors (rhomboid major, rhomboid minor and trapezius).
- Chin tuck (seated or lying) to lengthen the cervical spine and reinforce optimal posture.

In 2003 the Parkinson's Disease Society developed an exercise programme called 'Keeping Moving'. The programme was developed as a group exercise, but a booklet and video are available to enable people to exercise independently (Parkinson's Disease Society 2004c). The programme aims to minimise musculoskeletal limitation and postural deformities and promote independence through the maintenance of functional capacity. The programme involves relaxation and an emphasis on slow, controlled movements synchronised with breathing, and elements of strengthening, balance, coordination and flexibility. Pilates and/or core stability trained exercise professionals will be familiar with the type of exercises within the programme. Examples of some of the exercises and the reasons for them are:

- Encourage backward chaining to get on and off the floor. This is a technique used by physiotherapists and postural stability exercise professionals to teach people how to get on and off the floor. It involves breaking the sequence into small component parts, teaching each part separately and arranging the parts sequentially.
- Pelvic tilt mobilises the pelvis and lumbar region, and encourages smooth, controlled movement. This is important for activities such as sit to stand and walking.
- Knee opening/knee drops develop trunk stability against limb loading and practise isolation and control of movement.
- Heel slides develop trunk stabilisation against limb loading and practise control and isolation of movement.
- Heel slide plus single arm pullover increases the complexity, controlling movements of opposing limbs.

Seated exercises:

- Sitting pelvic tilt to progress the lying pelvic tilt and practise it in a more functional position.
- Trunk rotations to increase range of movement and improve balance and co-ordination.

Standing exercises:

- Weight transference in standing position with both feet in contact with the floor. Encourage forward and backward sway that is gradually reduced until weight is appropriately balanced and steady. This can help with the weight transference needed for activities such as sit to stand and can help improve postural control and balance.

- Standing rotation to progress the seated version by maintaining upright standing posture.

(Ramaswany and Webber 2003.)

Postural instability Not everyone with PD will fall, but as the condition progresses the risk of a fall increases. There are several factors that contribute to falls, including the physical problems related to PD, ageing, the effects of medication and the environment. People often develop a kyphotic standing posture, with rigidity in the neck and shoulders spreading to the trunk and extremities. This stooping position and change in muscle tone places the individual at an increased risk of falling. Rigidity or contraction of the calf muscle can make it difficult to dorsiflex the foot, hindering a normal heel–toe walking action. This results in a shuffling type of gait with short steps. Rigidity around the ankle joint can eventually lead to walking on the balls of the feet, reducing the ability of the feet to absorb shock adequately and exacerbating balance problems. A client with postural instability may benefit from a targeted programme with specific fall-management strategies such as gait, dynamic posture, balance and functional floor activities to improve confidence and coping skills. Other approaches such as Alexander technique and tai chi may also contribute to improved balance and gait (Parkinson's Disease Society 2005a).

Strategies to prevent falls

- Encourage client to focus on one activity and move slowly, to compensate for the body's inability to respond automatically.
- Avoid turning too quickly; don't turn on the spot; walk in a half circle; take more steps.
- Be aware of activities that increase the risk of falling such as stepping backwards or reaching for something while walking.

- Try to swing arms and lengthen stride when walking.
- Encourage upright posture and looking ahead.
- Practice striking the ground heel first.
- Encourage client to avoid doing too many things at once such as walking and talking and/or carrying objects.
- Encourage client to take time to perform activities that involve changing positions, e.g. to sit on the side of the bed for a while before getting out of bed. This is particularly important if client feels light-headed.
- Only perform floor-based exercises if clients can get themselves up off the floor.
- Check that any walking aid used has been recommended by a physiotherapist, as some walking aids may not be appropriate for people with PD and actually increase the risk of tripping or falling.
- Use a solid support such as a wall for standing exercises, especially for activities like calf raises that require balance.
- Ensure close supervision for balance exercises and gait training.
- Footwear with rubber soles tend to grip the floor and may cause a trip.
- Ensure a safe, clutter-free exercise environment to minimise the risk of trips and falls.

(Parkinson's Disease Society 2003.)

Freezing

People with PD can also have problems with 'freezing'. When this happens people feel as though their feet are stuck to the ground, even though their upper body wants to move forward. This causes them to stop suddenly. Freezing often occurs when people are approaching doorways and narrow spaces. It is also more likely to occur when people are feeling anxious or are in crowded places or unfamiliar situations. Changes in the surface such as moving to an uneven surface or a different pattern on a carpet can also cause a freeze. It can also happen when trying to initiate other movements, such as getting out of bed, lifting a cup to drink or stepping off after getting up from a sitting position. This is sometimes referred to as 'start hesitation' (Parkinson's Disease Society 2003a). The problems involved with initiating movement and freezing may leave people feeling unsteady on their feet and at an increased risk of falls.

Practical ways of helping with freezing There are a variety of methods that people find help them overcome 'freezing' and different methods will work for different people. If you are working with a client with PD, find out what works for them and if there is anything you can do to assist. Try not to distract the person when they are walking, as this will affect their concentration. The following cues can be used to help initiate and maintain movement and can be helpful for people experience freezing:

- **Proprioceptive cues, e.g. weight shift method** Instead of trying to move forward, focus on shifting the weight from one leg to the other as this can sometimes make it easier to step forward. Taking a step back before walking forward may also help. However, these methods may not be appropriate if balance is a problem.
- **Visual cues** Some people find it helps to identify a definite target and walk towards it. Stepping over a mark on the floor can help, or dropping a piece of paper and stepping over it. Other people find that trying to step over an imaginary obstacle can help initiate movement.
- **Auditory cues** Decide which leg to move first and then say '1, 2, 3, step' or 'ready, steady, go'. The client or the person with the client can say this. Counting from one to 10 while walking or using a marching rhythm or a small metronome are methods that work for different people.

• **Cognitive cues** Some people find it helpful to memorise parts of a movement sequence, mentally rehearsing a movement or visualising the length of a step.

Communication

An inability to use facial expressions and changes in speech such as rhythm, rate and intonation can have a big impact on communication for people with PD. Communication problems can lead to withdrawal and isolation so it is important for the exercise professional to be aware of these difficulties. Try to avoid making assumptions about how a person is feeling or their ability to understand based on body language, gesture and facial expression. Allow more time, and try to find ways to enhance communication (Parkinson's Disease Society 2003*b*).

Guidelines for exercise

• Timing of an exercise will be influenced by a number of factors. People who are on medication will know when it is working well, and whether they feel well enough to exercise.
• It is not appropriate to exercise if the client is feeling tired, if there has been a change in medication or if there has been a worsening of symptoms.
• Don't make assumptions about what a person can or cannot do.
• Teach transitions carefully, taking into account postural hypotension.
• Break down complex movement sequences into smaller components.
• Encourage people to practise exercises at a conscious level. This approach is used in exercises such as Pilates, where the mind–body connection is a key principle.
• Use a range of visual, auditory or proprioceptive cues to help people initiate and maintain movement, and to facilitate learning.
• Take into account co-morbidities such as heart disease.
• Only work within your own levels of competence and confidence. Seek advice where appropriate.
• Be sensitive to possible increased levels of frustration and depression that people with PD may experience.
• Provide appropriate support to help clients continue with the programme, such as telephone calls, an inclusive environment and social support (family and friends).

Table 13.5	Summary of exercise guidelines for Parkinson's disease		
Training guidelines	*Cardiovascular*	*Muscle strength*	*Flexibility*
Frequency	Structured exercise 3 times a week minimum. ADL and leisure activities can be carried out on non-exercise days.	2–3 non-consecutive days a week	5–7 days a week
Intensity	No consensus on optimal intensity. Moderate intensity may be appropriate 55–70	No consensus on optimal intensity. Initiate programme at low levels of	To the point of mild tension but not to pain or discomfort.

Table 13.5	Summary of exercise guidelines for Parkinson's disease cont.		
Training guidelines	Cardiovascular	Muscle strength	Flexibility
Intensity cont.	per cent of HRmax. Some people may need to initiate a programme at lower levels of intensity.	intensity using light resistance.	
Time	30 min. This can be broken down into smaller bouts e.g. 3 x 10 min.	I set of 8–12 reps	Hold stretch for 20–30 sec. Repeat each stretch 2–5 times.
Type	Arm or leg ergometry, walking, rowing, water-based.	8–10 exercises including major muscle groups. Fixed equipment may provide more support. Emphasis on erector spinae, rhomboids, middle and lower trapezius, gastrocnemius and quadriceps. Include functional activities such as sit to stand, squats and step-ups.	Static stretching is appropriate for people with mild muscle tightness. General stretching programme with an emphasis on increasing ROM in muscles which promote extension of the spine, hips and knees, and rotation of the spine.

Neuromuscular
Postural and balance exercises to improve the mind–body connection and encourage smooth, controlled movement (Ramaswany and Webber 2003). As the disease progresses, a more specialised programme with an emphasis on transfers, balance and gait will be necessary.

ACSM (2005*b*); Protas and Stanley (2003).

SUPPORTING CLIENTS TO CHANGE EXERCISE BEHAVIOUR

PART **FOUR**

This section of the book describes a way of working with referred clients to assist with the process of change and develop motivation towards adherence to an activity/exercise programme. It discusses how to create a helping relationship, focusing on how to work in a client-centred way using an empathetic, non-judgemental and relational style. It also explores one model of behaviour change, which can be used to increase the instructor's awareness of the processes people move through when undertaking change, and discusses strategies for assisting with the management of behaviour, thoughts and feelings in relation to the change process.

CREATING A HELPING RELATIONSHIP

14

The role of the personal trainer

The role of the personal trainer is to work with clients and enable and empower them to make their own decisions about the life changes that most enhance their health and well-being. The role includes:

- initial assessment and information gathering;
- negotiating a working contract;
- establishing a working alliance;
- building rapport and relationship.

In the initial stages the focus is on making contact with the client and gathering information to assess her or his needs, awareness and readiness to make changes; commitment to undertaking the personal work needed to make the changes; self-efficacy and belief about her or his ability to make these changes; and negotiating a provisional contract of working to enable successful change.

As the relationship and working alliance develops, the role of the trainer may diversify; s/he may need to:

- provide information (teacher);
- actively listen (counsellor);
- offer different strategies and interventions (creative and strategic planner);
- offer motivation and support (nurturer and supporter);
- help clients to establish goals (goal-setter);
- challenge clients and test/check their reality, perception, beliefs (liberator).

The quality of the relationship that develops between client and trainer is one of the most important factors for contributing towards effective longer-term changes implemented by the client.

Initial assessment and information gathering

Prior to devising an exercise and activity programme it is essential to find out about the client's lifestyle. (Refer to Chapter 4.)

The working contract

The provisional assessment enables the first steps towards building an effective working relationship with the person. It also enables a working contract to be developed. The duration of specific working contracts will be affected by the employment contract within the specific organisation. Some will offer short-term support working with direct help through a specific time period, others will provide longer-term support, depending on the set-up of any specialist schemes that operate in the organisation and whether they have the support of funding and/or expertise from other local organisations (for example primary care trusts, mental health groups, etc.).

Short-term contracts In many referral services a short-term contract of working is all that is available. The disadvantage of short-term contracts is that they demand a more directive way of working, for example the inclusion of specific cognitive and behavioural change techniques and strategies to promote self-management and self-help. These strategies are very effective and a directive approach works well for some people, but for others it can feel too imposed and paternalistic, which in the longer term may decrease the person's adherence and success at making changes.

Longer-term contracts In some services, there might be the opportunity to work with clients on a longer-term contract. An advantage of longer-term contracts is that the trainer can develop a deeper working alliance with the client and operate in a more exploratory and experimental way. The process of helping a client to make changes can include:

- identifying and exploring blocks to success as they present (for example relapses);
- encouraging an exploratory and creative attitude to confronting and managing these blocks and learning about the self;
- supporting the client as they work through these blocks and towards their goals.

Shorter-term working contracts will also enable the above to some extent. However, with a longer-term contract the relationship between the trainer and client can deepen (more empathy, attunement, positive regard, etc.). A longer-term contract can also offer more support to the person as they struggle to implement the changes they desire, providing the trainer with a greater understanding of the person. Longer-term working may help the client to access and sustain the level of motivation they need to maintain the changes more permanently.

In reality, a lifetime of choosing unhealthy behaviours and habits and the beliefs and attitudes the person holds that support these beliefs are unlikely to change overnight.

The working alliance

Establishing a relationship and developing a working alliance are also priorities as they influence the quality and level of the work undertaken. It is essential that the helper is able to reflect on action (look back at the effective-

ness of the interventions made after working with the client at each session and at the end of the work), and also in action (being aware of the effectiveness of interventions during their work with the client) (Boud et al.1985). The trainer will also need to be able to adapt his or her working style to suit different client needs. Some clients may need a more directive approach at times (being guided towards what to do); others will need a more exploratory approach, where they can experiment with different changes and decide which changes suit them and their lifestyle. Some clients need lots of support and encouragement and may be more dependent on specific support interventions, while others will be more inclined towards self-management and will only need occasional reassessments to discuss their progress and are happier being left to get on with things. It is essential that the trainer is reflective and creative so that s/he can adapt his or her way of working to accommodate different needs.

When the trainer's work with the client is due to end, s/he should review progress with the client and identify how s/he intends to move forward into self-management. Any additional support that is available should be pointed out (re-referral). Identify coping strategies that the client has established to manage change (internal and external support systems etc.). In addition, all records of information that relate to the work with the client should be stored securely and maintained for future reference.

Building rapport and relationship

The relationship developed between a client and the health professionals working with the client is one of the most important factors to promote growth and development. In his report discussing ways of working with obesity, Waine (2002) recommends a 'patient-centred approach' that emphasises compassion and appropriate use of communication skills, relational skills and intimacy for helping individuals to manage obesity. A relational approach like this is proposed as a way of working with all persons referred to exercise and activity to assist with the management of their condition.

Waine recommends that the approach should be:

- empathic, as opposed to unconcerned, about the person's struggles in relation to their condition;
- unbiased, as opposed to judgemental, about the person. This includes being aware of any prejudgements, self-righteousness and blame regarding the person's contribution to and responsibility for their condition from their behaviour choices (inactivity, smoking, alcohol, poor eating habits, etc.);
- supportive, as opposed to dismissive;
- accepting, as opposed to finding fault and blaming;
- optimistic, as opposed to sceptical, highlighting the positive changes that can be made by simple and achievable adjustments and the positive impact that each small change can make.

The core conditions

The client-centred (or patient-centred) approach evolves from the work of humanistic therapist Carl Rogers. Rogers (Rogers and Stevens 1967: 90) asserted that the client is the best expert on him- or herself and is capable of working out the solutions to his or her problems in the right environment or climate. He suggested that a climate where the core conditions were present was enough for the person to grow, develop and reach full potential. The three primary core conditions for building a positive relationship to bring about successful change are:

- congruency (being one's whole self, honestly, without putting on a front or a facade/mask);
- empathy (being able to see things from the other's perspective, putting oneself in the other person's position);
- unconditional positive regard (feeling a sense of warmth for the struggles the person presents).

Congruency

Congruency is being totally honest and genuine in the relationship. The helper needs to be aware of the thoughts and feelings going on within him- or herself, and be able to be manage these feelings without denying or discounting them, and be able to communicate them, if appropriate.

Most people are able to sense incongruence, when someone is putting on a front to perform a role. People can also recognise when someone is not communicating genuine thoughts or feelings, and consequently will often hold back from revealing themselves at any deeper level. It is worth noting that 55 per cent of our communication comes from body language, 38 per cent from voice tone and 7 per cent from the words we use. Clearly, any discrepancy between what we say and how we feel will be communicated at some level. The response we get may actually tell us more about what we are communicating than what we say or how we say it.

Similarly, with a person who is unafraid to be who s/he is, others are more likely to develop trust and consequently reveal more of themselves. However, it is essential not to just 'blurt out impulsively every feeling and accusation under the comfortable impression that one is being genuine' (Rogers and Stevens 1967: 91) as this is not helpful! The key is to be aware and recognise one's own inner responses and to process them in a way that is sensitive to the helping relationship.

An example: working with a client who frequently relapses from the activity plan To deny or ignore any feeling of frustration, disappointment or intolerance you may be feeling inside may be missing an opportunity to gather some key information about what the client may actually be feeling about her- or himself. Awareness of one's own internal processes can often enable more effective inquiry about the client's experience. One's feelings can be communicated and worked with respectfully by asking: 'How do you feel about your relapse?' This may open the client to discussion of a series of events that proved to be a block to their activity programme, which may offer reasons for their relapse that can be worked with. The inquiry may also reveal that the client felt frustration and disappointment with him- or herself. Enabling this level of openness can provide the helper with an opportunity to show that these feelings are a natural response. The helper could then make an intervention that enables the person to recognise the *inner judge*, the aspect of oneself that likes to criticise and focus on the negative, and the *inner nurturer*, the aspect of oneself that is able to see the positive steps and focus on these, so validating oneself (Stewart and Joines 1987). Raising awareness of these aspects of the self can be used to help balance any inner conflicts and move the client towards becoming his or her own best friend.

Empathy

Empathy is the ability to see things from the other person's perspective, to put yourself into his or her position and understand his or her world as if it were your own, without losing the 'as if' quality (Rogers and Stevens 1967: 93). In order to do this we need to be aware of any prejudices and closed-mindedness within us and put these issues to one side. We also need to be able to sideline any need to analyse and evaluate, which only helps us see the other people's worlds from *our* perspective, not theirs! Removing these barriers to intimacy will help to minimise projection of our own issues into the client's world. Erskine (1999) proposes the idea of moving beyond empathy by using inquiry and questioning skills that enable the person to tell her or his own story.

An example: working with the client who frequently relapses from his or her activity plan   A personally empathetic response from an instructor might be to state: 'I feel disappointed and frustrated with myself.' This type of response, though sometimes useful in that it might help the client to contact denied feelings in her- or himself, actually describes more of the helper's world and perspective than it does of the client's. A better response would be to ask how the relapse made the client feel. This enables the client to use his or her own voice and describe his or her own feelings in response to the situation, which gives a truer picture of the world as s/he sees and experiences it.

Rogers (Rogers and Stevens 1967: 93) quotes: 'If I am truly open to the way life is experienced by another person – if I can take his world into mine – then I run the risk of seeing life in his way, of being changed myself, and we all resist change. So we tend to view this other person's world only in our terms, not in his. We analyse and evaluate it. We do not understand it. But when someone understands how it feels and seems to be me, without wanting to analyse me or judge me, then I can blossom and grow in that climate.'

To demonstrate empathy in a relationship demands a number of skills, the primary one being the ability to listen actively with attunement to what the other person is saying. These skills are discussed further under the heading 'Interpersonal skills'.

Unconditional positive regard

Unconditional positive regard is about showing respect and warmth for the people with whom you are working. It is about prizing them as individuals in their own right, with their own unique way of being and valuing who they are without making judgements or decisions that they should be any other way.

An example: working with the person who constantly relapses from her or his intended exercise plan This person may stir up feelings of frustration, which might raise judgements inside the helper. These feelings need to be acknowledged within the helper as an aspect of themselves and processed as a personal response. It may be that the client is experiencing the same or similar feelings about him- or herself; this can be explored by inquiring: 'How do you feel when you relapse?' The client may then acknowledge these or similar feelings and the process can move on by the helper asking: 'How can we work together to move through this barrier?' Unconditional positive regard is about accepting the whole person and respecting the self s/he are presenting as an aspect of the person. It is about accepting his or her humanness and the difficulties s/he may experience and the effect this has on his or her life and self-esteem. It is fairly normal for human beings to dislike and judge certain human behaviours and to have prejudices. However, in order to demonstrate unconditional positive regard one needs to be aware of these and take responsibility for these judgements as one's own. They should not be used to condemn or disempower the other person.

Carl Rogers believed that applying these core conditions to a helping relationship would help the person develop a strong enough sense of self to move forward and make changes.

As personal trainers we need to recognise that while we have certain pieces of knowledge the client needs, it is the client who knows his or her lifestyle and what changes will work for him or her in life. Resistance to our 'useful' suggestions should be acknowledged as an indicator that somehow this advice is not right for this client. A more effective approach than giving specific advice (Do this! Do that!) is to explore the client's world and his or her way of operating and identify a range of potential ways that s/he can work with to move towards making the desired changes. Relapse can be viewed as acknowledgement that the approach selected was not the 'best fit' for the client, and allows other ways of making changes to be explored. The key is to be creative and work with the client, helping her or him to choose approaches to change that work personally rather than imposing specific programmes. This way of working does not necessarily provide the quick fix, if indeed there is such a thing, but it is a way of working that enables effective change in the longer term.

Motivational interviewing techniques

Motivational interviewing is a client-centred method of gathering information to explore a client's readiness to change. It can be used to elicit information about the client's concerns about specific areas of his or her life that s/he would like to change. This information can then be used to discuss with the person the advantages and disadvantages of making the changes proposed. The information collected can also indicate where the client is in relation to the 'cycle of change' model (contemplating, preparing, action) and can identify his or her personal levels of motivation, any support systems in place and any resistance or ambivalence to making changes. It can also help the personal trainer to provide the appropriate support and intervention to help the client make a positive decision for her- or himself. Finally, it enables the personal trainer to negotiate goals and strategies to work towards with the client.

Focusing on the client During any assessments with the client, it is important to make him or her the most important person in the room and demonstrate this by:

• facing forwards and looking at him or her;

- removing any barriers such as desks;
- being interested and attentive to what s/he is saying;
- being sensitive to your own facial expressions and body language;
- minimising distractions by using a private room, placing a 'do not disturb' sign on the door and ensuring mobile phones are switched off;
- leaning forwards slightly – but not so far that you appear aggressive;
- keeping an open body and upright posture that is comfortable but not too stiff;
- maintaining eye contact without staring;
- reflecting warmth by demonstrating the core conditions (empathy, unconditional positive regard, congruence);
- smiling naturally and being present for the client;
- avoiding fidgeting.

Communication skills

Questioning

Asking appropriate questions can be an effective method for gathering information from the client. However, there can sometimes be a tendency to ask too many questions, which may block some clients from speaking if they feel they are under interrogation. Asking too many questions may also prevent active listening to what the client is saying, because the trainer may be focused more on asking the questions than really listening and hearing the client's responses.

There are different types of questions that personal trainers and fitness instructors can use to gather information from their clients. Questioning is a method of inquiry that can enable the trainer/helper to gain a fuller picture of the person's subjective experience.

Open questions

These are most effective for gathering information in greater depth. They are questions that begin with the words: What? Who? How? Where? Why? When? These types of question, when asked in the presence of the core conditions, will generally enable the client to relax and encourage her or him to speak openly. Examples of such questions are: 'How did you feel when you heard about your diagnosis?', 'How did you feel when you broke from your diet?', 'Would you like to explore that further?'

Further information can be gathered from open questioning by using **probing questions** to encourage the client to expand on his or her initial response; or by using **focusing questions** to inquire more closely about a specific response that may help to define the problem more clearly. For example:

Probing: 'Could you explain that?', 'Tell me more about that,' 'Have you ever experienced that sensation before?'

Focusing: 'Tell me more about the pain in your joint', 'Where exactly are you feeling the discomfort?' 'What does that sensation feel like?'

Active listening

Listening and hearing what the client is saying is a real skill and requires practice and much empathy on behalf of the trainer. It also requires the presence of the other core conditions, unconditional positive regard and congruence. Active listening can be demonstrated in the following ways:

- Making some acknowledgement as the client speaks, for example: nodding the head, making eye contact, or saying 'yes' or another sound (ummm, uh huh, etc.) that emphasises that they are being heard.
- Summarising what the client has said using

your own language, and using a questioning style so that they are able to correct anything misheard. For example: 'Am I hearing you say that you feel anxious when this happens?'
- Reflecting back what the client says by reading between the lines. For example: Client: 'and the doctors are just so insensitive,' Helper: 'Seeing other patients with cancer as you travelled with them made you feel scared?' Client: 'Yes.'

- Asking questions if you do not understand or if you need further information from what the client is saying, for example: 'Would you tell me more about that so I can get a better picture?'

Other barriers to listening, and ineffective questioning styles, are discussed in the *Complete Guide to Exercising Away Stress*, (Lawrence 2005).

MODEL OF BEHAVIOUR CHANGE

15

The trans-theoretical model of change

This is ONE model used for behaviour change. It provides a number of stages that relate to where an individual may be positioned in relation to the change process. Identifying the position of an individual in the cycle of change can help to identify appropriate strategies to assist with helping the individual to make positive changes. Fig. 15.1 provides a diagram of the trans-theoretical model of change.

Figure 15.1 Trans-theoretical model of change

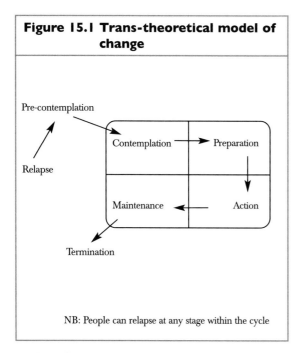

NB: People can relapse at any stage within the cycle

NB: Examples of dialogues at each stage of the change process are provided in the *Complete Guide to Exercising Away Stress,* Lawrence (2005).

Stages of change and interventions

Pre-contemplation

At this stage of the change cycle the individual is not aware s/he has a problem and is not thinking about making any changes. There may be resistance to the change process due to feelings of powerlessness or helplessness or possibly because of a fear of failure. At this stage the personal trainer can provide information that may assist the person to move closer towards contemplating making a change. They can give information in the form of handouts and leaflets that can help raise the client's awareness to the risks associated with continuing their existing behaviour. They can also use sensitive motivational interviewing techniques in a supportive and non-judgemental environment, which can encourage the client to explore any resistance and fears s/he may hold in relation to making a change in behaviour. Validating the client's feelings is important at this stage. Whatever a person feels is real for him or her, and these feelings will continually be a barrier to making changes unless they are acknowledged, accepted and managed.

The client's body language and non-verbal language can often provide an indication to defences and barriers that they are experiencing. The personal trainer can use open questioning techniques to inquire about the signs that the client is providing, if it seems appropriate for them to do so.

Contemplation

At this stage of the change process the individual is aware that a problem exists and is

Table 15.1 Decisional balance sheet	Advantages	Disadvantages
Change		
No change		

seriously considering making changes. S/he may experience internal conflicts regarding the advantages and disadvantages of making changes and may become stuck at this stage and move no further unless specific interventions are applied.

The personal trainer can help the client to explore the advantages and disadvantages of both changing, and not changing and also explore the risk and harm caused by the existing behaviour. This can be done using the decisional balance sheet outlined in table 15.1.

Cognitive dissonance

Using the decisional balance sheet can help to identify any inconsistency in the client and inner conflict between attitudes and behaviour. The trainer can raise awareness of these inner conflicts and encourage the client to explore them in an appropriate setting (counselling). One example might be a client who on the one hand is proactive towards banning things that pollute the atmosphere, and on the other hand smokes. These discrepancies could be pointed out to the client.

Another example might be that the client is wanting to make a change but at the same time fearful about it and feels s/he will not be able to succeed. One intervention could be to raise awareness of the very real fear that smoking is

a high contributory factor to CHD; however, this can sometimes trigger more fear and may encourage an anxious person to smoke even more, particularly if it is deeper feelings of fear that trigger the person to smoke. Another intervention could be to explore the fear that surrounds both polarities in thinking. Again this would require the skilled interventions of a counsellor, as these issues need to be dealt with sensitively and empathetically, as they are very real to the client's experience.

Any decision or choice to make changes ultimately lies with the client. It is not the role of the trainer to try and enforce specific changes, for even if the person complies with these changes in the short term, he or she is unlikely to do so in the long term. Attempting to coerce people to make the changes they are resisting is assuming they are not able to make effective choices for themselves. The issue here is that some of the choices people make are not the most effective for their health. However, to reiterate a point, the decision to change lies with the person, not with the instructor. If the client is contemplating making a change it is essential to promote the benefits of the change without dictating to build her or his commitment and confidence and reinforce her or his ability to do it; that there is a way and that s/he can manage the internal conflict and make the changes s/he desires.

It is also worthwhile for the trainer to encourage the client to use a diary to explore his or her behaviour. By keeping a diary the client will become more aware of things that might stop them from making changes. For example: 'I didn't go to the gym because I felt too tired. When I felt stressed I had another cup of coffee and a cigarette.' Keeping a diary can raise awareness of the client's behaviour and provide her or him with greater insight into ways s/he could make changes that are comparatively simple and easy. The trainer can point out these simpler ways and identify how much easier they would be to make. For example: a client who eats more junk food when s/he is stressed can be reminded that s/he could eat other foods that are more nutritious and would also help with his or her other goal of losing weight. A client who wants to stop smoking could become aware of when s/he smokes and other strategies could be implemented, such as taking a few deep breaths or doing something else before having a cigarette. It may be that these techniques eventually distract the person from thinking about smoking.

Preparation

At this stage of the change process the individual is ready to change and may have already made some small changes. They may have started using a diary to record their behaviours. They may have started a yoga class to help release stress, or reduced their coffee intake during the day. However, they are still not fully committed to the change process as yet.

The personal trainer can help at this stage by exploring a variety of options to bring about the desired changes and can speak with the client to strengthen his or her commitment and build confidence about making small changes. The trainer can help the client to set some small goals using the SMART method and establish an action plan for achieving these goals.

Action

At this stage of the change process the individual is making changes and has committed some time and energy to doing so. S/he may have made the changes for just one day or up to six months.

The personal trainer can help at this stage by focusing on the client's successes and positively affirming progress. This positive reinforcement helps to maintain motivation and can build self-efficacy and help the client to stay committed. The trainer can also guide the client towards using positive affirmations that will help the client maintain motivation and self-belief.

The trainer can also explore external stimuli that might trigger the behaviour and look at ways of avoiding or managing these stimuli (stimulus control). For example: a smoker may wish to avoid going to the bar after work where s/he will be tempted to have a cigarette. An alternative behaviour could be proposed, such as attending an exercise session or any other activity that will distract from the stimulus.

The trainer could suggest that the client has a massage or another personal reward for maintaining a change of behaviour. S/he can also explore the client's feelings about the change and encourage the client to look at the positive impact of her or his new behaviour. For example: a client who is new to exercise could be encouraged to consider how s/he feels better after the exercise session, even though s/he feels tired before s/he attends. This exploration of both the positive and negative aspects of the change can provide reinforcement that helps to maintain and manage the change of behaviour.

It can also be useful to explore a range of alternative behaviours and other coping strategies. For example: a client who drinks a cup of coffee when s/he is stressed could explore the option of drinking another beverage that will not trigger an additional stress response. S/he could also look at taking five minutes at intervals throughout the day to complete some desk exercises that can help reduce muscle tension. These alternatives provide new and different responses to the stimulus or trigger (counter-conditioning), a strategy that can help one to manage stress more positively. It is also useful to have a contingency plan to help the client maintain motivation when tempted to relapse.

Maintenance

At this stage of the change process the individual is sustaining the changes and preventing relapse. The new habit may be established and some coping strategies will already be in place for managing problem situations and avoiding temptation.

The role of the personal trainer now is to provide a helpful and supportive relationship and reinforce the positive behaviour by giving plenty of praise and encouragement, which acts as a reward and can help to increase the client's self-efficacy. The client will also need reminding of all her or his successes to help maintain motivation. S/he will also need to be made aware of possible cues that may indicate the likelihood of a relapse and have strategies in place to manage a relapse.

It may be worthwhile educating the client in how his or her thought processes might respond in times of relapse. Some clients will **overgeneralise** and see the slip as meaning a complete failure. Others may experience **selective abstraction**, where they focus only on the failure and not on any of the successes. Other clients will take **excessive responsibility** for the slip and see it as their own personal weakness. Others will **catastrophise**, go totally overboard, and exaggerate how bad the slip was.

Some clients use a mixture or even all of these thought processes to throw themselves out of the change cycle.

It is useful if the trainer can work with the client to help him or her recognise where potential slips may be attributed. For example: a client who sees a slip as a personal lack of will-power will experience a reduction in self-efficacy and personal power if they relapse, whereas a client who believes a slip is just a temporary lack of coping will maintain self-efficacy and is more likely to get back into the cycle. It is therefore useful if the trainer works with the client and explains that slips are often a natural occurrence until a new habit or change of behaviour is imprinted. It is worth recognising that even changing the way we think is a challenge for most people. For example, if one has spent 30–40 years thinking self-critical or negative thoughts then it will be a big challenge to break that behaviour pattern. A client who has smoked for 20 years will have an equal challenge to break a number of behaviour patterns that include buying cigarettes, lighting them, the hand-to-mouth action, the inhaling, etc. There are many behaviours that would have to change and each step the client makes is a success! It is essential to highlight all of these.

Relapse

At this stage of the cycle of change the client would have returned to his or her old behaviour. For example, s/he may have stopped exercising, returned to old eating or lifestyle patterns, started smoking again, etc. Relapse is a very uncomfortable experience for people who are trying to make changes, as it increases feelings of failure and hopelessness, which discourages them and makes them lose confidence and belief in their ability to make these changes: their self-efficacy.

The trainer can give support and encouragement and explore possible causes for the relapse. S/he can then review the client's action plan and work with the client to help him or her to re-enter the change cycle.

Termination

The new behaviour would be permanent at this stage and the client would have achieved his or her goal.

It usually takes clients a few attempts to move through the change cycle, and they experience a few relapses before reaching this stage. The change process in reality is not orderly; people get stuck at specific stages a few times before they achieve a permanent change of behaviours and habits.

The model represents the different levels of psychological functioning which interrelate and which require work to help the person make the desired changes. These are:

- presenting problem (the behaviour);
- negative thought processes (thinking);
- interpersonal difficulties (relationship with others);
- social/systemic difficulties (relationship with systems);
- intrapersonal difficulties (relationship with self).

The personal trainer can recognise where the person is within the cycle of change and this will help him or her to identify appropriate interventions s/he is qualified to manage, and also where his or her expertise ends and additional professional support, such as counselling, may be needed.

The personal trainer can help with the behavioural and to some extent the thinking levels of functioning. S/he would not be professionally qualified to deal with interpersonal, social or intrapersonal conflicts or difficulties the client may be experiencing. This highlights the importance of working with other professionals in a multi-discipline team to manage the change process effectively. Contacts for sources of further help are provided at the end of this book.

STRATEGIES FOR MAKING AND MANAGING CHANGES

16

The way a trainer works with a client will be dependent on a number of factors, which include:

Case conceptualisation How the trainer conceptualises and understands what the client presents (physical/medical conditions, mental/emotional state, beliefs, attitudes etc.) and the trainer's attunement and empathy to the client's experience.

The working contract negotiated In many referral services a short-term contract of working is all that is available. This, in many ways, demands that a more directive approach to working with the client is taken; for example, selecting specific cognitive and behavioural change techniques and strategies that promote self-management and self-help. In some services, the opportunity to work with clients on a longer-term contract may be available. The advantage of this is that there is the potential for the trainer to develop a deeper working alliance with the client and use more exploratory and experimental methods, identifying and examining blocks to success as they present, encouraging an exploratory and creative attitude to confronting and managing these blocks and supporting clients as they work towards their goals.

The working alliance The duration, intimacy and commitment to the relationship and work undertaken will also affect the approach the trainer uses to help the client. For example, a client who has been working for a longer time and who has made some successful changes will require a different approach from a client who has just been referred and has yet to start making the necessary changes.

The client's readiness to change Identifying where a client is in relation to the model of change will also influence the strategies the trainer uses, as will the client's self-efficacy and belief in her or his own ability to make these changes.

Raising awareness to assist with change

Prochaska and Diclemente name ten common processes that people involved in a change and growth process move through. Some helpful strategies that can be applied are listed under each of these processes (cited by P. Jackson, in Feltham and Horton 2000: 400).

Consciousness-raising and self-monitoring

These are methods for gathering information about oneself and one's problem(s) and monitoring and raising awareness of circumstances that trigger specific lifestyle choices. They include:

- keeping a diary to monitor eating patterns (type of food, time of day, quantity, mood etc.);
- keeping a diary to monitor smoking or alcohol (when, where, mood, thoughts, etc.);
- keeping a diary to monitor emotions and thoughts (when, where, who with, doing what, etc.);
- keeping a record of daily activity levels (how long, how hard, what type, when, etc.);
- keeping an exercise log (frequency, intensity, time, type, etc.);

- writing a hassle list for all the things that add to stress levels (what, when, where, etc.);
- researching a medical condition;
- researching the effects of prescribed medications;
- researching ways for managing a condition.

Self-liberation

One takes a positive approach and believes in the possibility of change and makes the choice to commit to take action. For example:

- using the decisional balance sheet to assist making the decision (for example weighing up the decision to become more active);
- finding the inner determination to commit to working with and handling the medical condition;
- using positive self-talk to maintain the self-belief that the condition can be managed.

Social liberation

This involves raising awareness of the increasing opportunity for alternative behaviours in society. For example:

- diabetes groups;
- cardiac rehabilitation programmes;
- GP referral exercise schemes;
- diet and exercise clubs;
- smoking cessation programmes etc.

Counter-conditioning

One introduces alternative behaviour to replace the specific problem behaviour. For example:

- take a few deep breaths instead of having a cigarette;
- go for a walk before sitting down in front of the television and having a drink;
- take five minutes to sit and meditate before starting and finishing the day to promote positive thinking.

Stimulus control

These techniques are used to reduce the stimuli that trigger specific behaviours, for example:

- putting cigarettes out of reach when driving;
- buying only healthy foods to keep at home;
- sitting down to eat at predetermined times rather than combining eating with other activities (e.g. while cooking in the kitchen);
- drinking water when hunger pangs occur;
- listening to a positive thinking tape to retrain negative thinking patterns;
- not visiting environments where the behaviour may be triggered (e.g. the pub).

Self re-evaluation

Evaluate how one thinks and feels about oneself in relation to the problem behaviour or medical condition. For example:

- speak to a therapist or counsellor regarding depression related to diagnosis of cancer or other life-threatening disease;
- keep a journal to recognise how one thinks about oneself in relation to a behaviour, e.g. 'When I get stressed I immediately raid the cupboards and binge. This makes me feel really bad and I end up berating myself and putting myself down.'

Environmental re-evaluation

Recognise how the problem behaviour affects the family, relatives, the wider community and the environment. For example:

- recognise that smoking may affect the health of babies and children;
- recognise how one's bad moods, negative thinking and unassertive behaviours impact others, which may in turn affect their behaviour;

- recognise the impact of depression on relationships with family and friends;
- recognise how the overuse of alcohol impacts others.

Contingency/reinforcement management

These techniques involve giving oneself a reward or a creature comfort when a single, small change has been made, for example managing smoking or eating behaviour successfully for a day. Rewards can include:

- small treats (a bubble bath, watching a favourite video, etc.);
- medium treats (buying a new outfit, a body massage, etc.);
- larger treats (a holiday or health spa retreat, etc.).

Dramatic relief

This involves experiencing and expressing feelings that may be linked with the problem behaviour and identifying possible solutions to manage these. For example:

- working with a counsellor or support worker to discuss feelings, for example clients diagnosed with a life-threatening illness may feel angry. It is essential that this anger is explored so that it is not focused inward towards the self (causing depression, addictive behaviours, etc.) or outwards in a way that could be destructive to supportive relationships;
- working with a personal trainer to identify exercises and other activities to find a physical release for feelings of anger;
- writing a journal to get the feelings out on paper and discussing these with a close friend or supportive family member;
- writing or drawing pictures to express feelings and again discussing these with a supportive

friend or family member (examples of creative activities to explore feelings are discussed in the *Complete Guide to Exercising Away Stress* (Lawrence 2005).

Helping relationships and support systems

Receiving appropriate support and encouragement is a key factor in assisting with the management of behaviour change. It is essential to have a support system of people who care and whom the client is able to trust to speak openly about the problems s/he may be experiencing. Support can come from a variety of sources:

- friends
- family
- partners
- personal trainers and fitness instructors
- health professionals/GPs
- counsellors, etc.
- church, mosque, or other spiritual community.

Some clients struggle with asking for help and support and others struggle with finding the support they need. Blocks that prevent a person from social interaction and support can include low self-esteem and self-belief, low assertiveness, depression and a habit of doing things alone. Clients need to be encouraged to build a support system proactively (calling friends, joining groups, etc.) and decreasing the number of activities they take part in alone (watching television, etc.).

Other techniques for assisting the change process

There is not one specific technique that works for all clients. It is the trainer's ability to be

197

perceptive and responsive to the client's needs that will enable her or him to make changes. As previously mentioned, the relationship developed between client and trainer is possibly one of the most important aspects for promoting change. Some clients will work more effectively with different relational styles and different approaches. Similarities between client and trainer may have a bearing on the effectiveness of specific interventions, for example matching of age, gender, ethnicity, and social class may all impact the relationship and the effectiveness of specific interventions.

For example, a male client may work better with a male trainer, an Asian client may work better with an Asian trainer, an older client may work better with an older trainer, a client from a working-class background may work better with a trainer from a working-class background. These elements of difference are often ignored, but they can make a significant difference to the effectiveness of specific interventions.

Modifying behaviour

These are techniques used for making conscious changes to habitual behaviour, and include:

- eating more slowly and more consciously;
- having short breaks while eating a meal;
- drinking single shots of alcohol rather than double shots;
- using mixers to dilute alcoholic drinks;
- taking a few deep breaths or going for a short walk before having a cigarette.

Goal-setting

Goal-setting techniques can be a positive way of making changes and establishing appropriate time-frames for getting things done. The **SMART** method can help to make goals workable:

- **S**pecific – decide what you want.
- **M**easurable – how will you know you are succeeding?
- **A**chievable – is your goal possible?
- **R**eward yourself – treat yourself as you achieve.
- **T**ime-framed – set time limits for goals.

Assertiveness training

Learning to become more assertive can help people raise their confidence levels and manage themselves and their lives more effectively (Lawrence 2005). Methods for developing assertiveness include:

- taking an assertiveness training course;
- reading an assertiveness book;
- personal counselling.

Positive-self talk and thinking strategies

These techniques promote awareness of how the mind works and are a key to making someone their own best friend (Lawrence 2005). For example:

- becoming aware of the inner dialogue and whether one's thoughts and beliefs are positive or negative;
- sitting for a short while to monitor one's thoughts;
- noticing the negative thoughts and words one uses to describe oneself, for example: 'I am so stupid … useless … no will-power … etc.';
- replacing negative thoughts with positive self-affirmations that validate the self, for example: 'I can handle this … I am worthwhile … I am valued,' etc.;
- listening to positive affirmation tapes;
- writing down several positive things about oneself on a daily basis.

Visualisation

Clients can use visualisation techniques to create picture images of their goals. Clients can be asked to:

- focus on their specific goals (e.g. move around without becoming breathless, performing a series of exercises or an exercise class with ease, seeing themselves eat healthier foods, lose weight, etc.);
- focus on themselves when they have achieved their goals (how they will move, look, feel, speak, walk, etc.);
- make the picture image brighter and bigger and add colour to make the picture more visual and alive in their minds;
- explore the thoughts and feelings they hold in relation to seeing themselves achieve this goal, which can be used to assist their motivation;
- connect these memories with a physical gesture (for example, touching the forefinger to the thumb). This connection can be used as a prompt for a daily meditation to remind them of their goals and to maintain focus. It can also be used as a prompt for when times are tough and they feel like giving up.

Visualisation techniques can also be used to decrease the vividness of less pleasant pictures clients might create about themselves. These pictures can be made smaller, darker and taken further away in the mind's eye.

Relaxation techniques

Relaxation techniques are ways of managing the physical symptoms of anxiety, stress and depression that may present in clients with specific medical conditions. A range of different relaxation techniques and relaxation scripts are provided in the *Complete Guide to*

Exercising Away Stress (Lawrence 2005). These include:

- active muscular relaxation;
- passive muscular relaxation;
- imagery/visualisation;
- the Benson method.

Promoting self-management for behaviour change

Encouraging a person to make the decision to change certain aspects of their lifestyle is a positive step, although it can also seem an unmanageable task for many. Sometimes the specific changes can feel very uncomfortable and unnatural and may provide the person with increased stress. Some keys to people making any successful change are:

- to empower them to make their own choices (whether you agree with them or not, they know what is right and works for them);
- to provide education and support them in their decisions (facilitating learning and exploring without dictating);
- encouraging them to take one step at a time and reflect and learn from their experiences (offering support and encouragement and not an 'I told you so', self-righteous attitude);
- engaging with and encouraging them to commit to a decision and process (listening to them and reading between the lines, checking their self-belief and readiness to make particular changes);
- encouraging them to keep going and never give up (developing their determination, self-belief and a positive mental attitude).

The following 10 steps can be used as a list of strategies to assist clients with managing their own change processes (e.g. increasing activity, changing lifestyle habits and eating patterns, etc.).

1. Make lists of all the things they would like to change.
2. Decide what changes are the most important for them.
3. Raise their awareness of the advantages and disadvantages of changing each behaviour and aspect.
4. Work out specific goals to create the changes they desire.
5. Get to know more about their own behaviour and the things they want to change by keeping a diary.
6. Identify what alternative strategies and behaviours they could use when the desire to relapse into old behaviour is triggered.
7. Prepare to make the changes.
8. Set the date when they will start making changes.
9. Be ready to cope with setbacks.
10. Stay motivated and keep getting support!

Step 1: Make lists of all the things clients would like to change

The first thing to explore is what clients would like to change. Exploring the current risks to their health and ways of making changes will help them decide what specifically they would like to change. The specific changes each person chooses will vary, but may include:

- increasing daily activity (walking to the shops instead of driving);
- starting an exercise programme (going to an exercise class);
- lowering stress levels (attending a relaxation class or listening to a relaxation tape before going to bed);
- giving up smoking or reducing their cigarette intake;
- drinking less alcohol;
- reducing the fat in their diet;
- eating more vegetables and fruit.

Step 2: Decide what changes are the most important to the client

It would be unwise to expect a person to change everything about her or his lifestyle overnight, although some people are able to do this. It is more realistic to take one or two things at a time and work on making changes to these before moving on to other areas.

Individuals need to be encouraged to prioritise the things they would like to change and select what seems to be the most appropriate thing for them. Some people like to succeed at managing the easier changes first as a way of boosting their confidence. Others will want to tackle the toughest challenge straight away. The key is for people to decide the right way for themselves.

Step 3: Raise clients' awareness of the advantages and disadvantages of changing their behaviour

A decisional balance sheet can be used to work out the advantages and disadvantages of making specific changes. This will identify factors that will affect the individual's commitment to the change process. It will also identify some of the specific blocks to that process.

Step 4: Work out specific goals for creating the changes they desire

Encourage clients to use the SMART method for setting their goals:

Specific – decide on goal.

Measurable – decide on measures that will indicate they are succeeding.

Achievable – check their goals are possible and realistic.

Activity to identify blocks

Take a blank piece of paper and ask clients to draw a pathway.
Ask them to write their goals at some point along the pathway.
Ask them to draw closed gates along the pathway to indicate all the blocks that may prevent them from being successful. A block could be a person, an occasion, a feeling or a thought process.
Take some time to explore with them ways of working to enable them to open these gates.
These may include:
Support from a friend;
Breathing exercises;
Listening to relaxation tapes;
Positive self-talk and affirmations.

Adapted from: *The Complete Guide to Exercising Away Stress*, Lawrence (2005.)

Rewards – identify a range of rewards that can be given as treats for making steps to achieve and manage change.

Time-framed – encourage clients to establish time-frames for specific goals and their review.

Step 5: Encourage clients to get to know more about their behaviour and lifestyle choices by keeping a diary

To promote successful change it is essential to know as much as possible about reasons for existing habits and behaviours. A diary can be used with people who want to become more active, people who want to change their eating habits, people who want to give up smoking and people who want to manage stress. The diary can be used to record thoughts, feelings, environment (where they are and who they are with) and what triggers them to make specific lifestyle choices/behaviours (smoking, eating junk food, etc.). Examples of layouts of a behaviour change diaries are provided in tables 16.1 and 16.2.

The key is for the person to record:

- **A**ntecedents – what happened before the behavior;
- **B**ehaviour – what behaviour was triggered;
- **C**onsequences – how they felt afterwards.

It is worth noting that while poor choices offer people temporary relief, if they are attempting to make changes to their lifestyle they may also trigger negative feelings such as guilt, shame, self-blame and self-disgust that can contribute to a relapse from the path of change. The role of the

Table 16.1	Example of behaviour change diary entry (1)		
Example	*Antecedent*	*Behaviour*	*Consequence*
Eating	Someone upset me, I feel alone and fed up	Ate biscuits	Feel more cheerful, comforted
Smoking	I got stuck in traffic	Lit up a cigarette	Feel more relaxed
Drinking	I got home from work tired	Had a glass of wine	Felt de-stressed
Inactivity	Had a long day at work, felt tired	Sat and watched TV instead of going for a walk	Feel relaxed

Table 16.2	Example of behaviour change diary entry (2)		
	Antecedent	*Behaviour*	*Consequence*
Morning: **11am**	Felt frustrated Was worrying about ...	Had a cigarette Ate biscuits	Felt relieved
Afternoon	Had argument with colleague	Ate junk food	Felt comforted
Evening	Felt relieved to be home from work	Ate planned healthier meal	Felt pleased with myself

trainer is to help clients explore these feelings (s/he might encourage work with a therapist or counsellor) and provide encouragement and support to enable them to get back into the change process.

Step 6: Identify what alternative strategies could be used when the old behaviour is triggered

The diary helps clients identify when they use old behaviours they want to change and when they use behaviours they may want to keep. A problem-solving approach can be used to identify both proactive and reactive strategies for coping when the desire to relapse presents.

Some pro-active (thinking ahead) strategies

Problem: Eating because feeling alone or fed up, instead:

- phone a friend and talk, share your feelings;
- go for a walk;
- join a group activity;
- eat a healthy snack.

Problem: Smoking when stuck in traffic, instead:

- have fruit or raw vegetables or mints in car instead of cigarette;

- put cigarettes out of reach;
- make a routine of taking deep breaths when in traffic.

Reactive strategies (thinking on your feet) are required when the behaviour is triggered unexpectedly. The positive aspect of this is that the more you have experimented with different ways of changing, the more you learn and the more reactive strategies you have available. For example:

- taking some deep breaths;
- using positive self-talk;
- removing yourself from the situation at a specific time and going for a walk;
- talking to a friend to manage the feelings.

When certain feelings are triggered it is an automatic response to reach for a known comfort aid or revert to the best-known way of coping. This is ok. The key is to encourage clients to learn from their experiences of relapse and get back on that wagon again, believing in their ability to make changes and adopting an 'I CAN DO IT' attitude, and the belief that they can make the changes they desire happen. This requires them to commit themselves fully to the process as a way of learning more about themselves, so they can help themselves and become their own best friend.

Problem-solving sheet

Encourage the client to explore the following on a sheet of paper:

1. What are the specific problems/triggers?
2. What are possible solutions for managing these triggers?
(Find as many as possible. You can ask friends or others to contribute their possible solutions. The range of solutions written down can also be childlike and although some may be inappropriate for real life practice (for example, stamping on the foot of someone who upsets you), these can still be effective ways for releasing emotions that contribute to triggering a specific behaviour, which in turn assist individuals with managing their response to the trigger.
3. Test the solutions
Encourage clients to become their own experiment and try different things.
4. Evaluate the results
Encourage clients to find out what works and what doesn't work for them and explore the reasons.
5. Repeat the process. Try another way of managing the behaviour and the triggers.

NB: Sometimes it is necessary to try out a few possible solutions to identify what works and what doesn't work and learn from the experience. There are always other solutions.

Step 7: Prepare them to make the specific changes

Once clients have identified what they want to change, what triggers old behaviour, and how much they indulge themselves in this behaviour (smoking, inactivity, etc.) they need to be encouraged to start building in small manageable changes using the following principles:

Frequency – how often
Intensity – the amount
Time – how long.

These principles are easier to use when planning activity; they can also be used to plan other changes of behaviour. See table 16.3 for an example.

Step 8: Set the date when they will start making changes

Encourage clients to make the commitment with themselves to start making changes. They can write this commitment down in a journal, share it with a friend or put a sticker on the fridge. The key is to make sure that whatever they have planned to do must be SMART and workable for them. Making short-term goals, medium-term goals and long-term goals will help them move towards the change they desire.

Step 9: Make sure they are ready to cope with set-backs

It is fairly common for things not to run exactly to plan. It is easier for clients to recover if they are prepared. They need to look at all the problem situations and blocks they have identified, and the strategies they have chosen to work with these blocks, and be ready to adopt alternative strategies.

Avoid complacency Educate clients so that they know missing one exercise session, having one cigarette or having a diet hiccup does not make a difference UNLESS it prevents them from starting again. If they relapse, encourage them to recommit to the change.

Beware of high-risk situations For

Table 16.3	The FIT principles of manageable change		
	Eating	*Drinking*	*Smoking*
Frequency	Eat take-out meals on fewer days of the week. Have a chocolate-free day.	Reduce the number of days on which you drink or go to pub. Have a drink-free day.	Reduce the number of cigarettes you smoke in one day. Have a smoke-free day.
Intensity	If you eat take-out meals choose a healthier option.	Reduce the quantity of alcohol you consume in one go. Have drinks with mixers so less alcohol is consumed.	Take fewer inhalations of each cigarette. Smoke a lighter brand. Use a cigarette filter.
Time	Eat more slowly. Take a break between courses so you allow yourself the experience of feeling full.	Go to the pub later in the day.	Delay each cigarette by 5–10 min.

some clients and some behaviours it may be easier to avoid certain situations. For example, a smoker may initially want to avoid situations where friends are smoking.

Be assertive Encourage clients to learn to say 'No thank you' if they are offered a cigarette or a cake. Encourage them to commit to their decision with power rather than saying, 'I'd love to, but …'

Coping with craving Encourage clients to be ready for strong urges that they will want to give in to. They do not last for long but can feel very intense. Educate them so that they are prepared and have strategies in place to deal with cravings, for example call a supportive friend when tempted.

Reward yourself Advise clients to plan a whole range of small rewards for each success. These could include a massage, a day at a health spa, a new outfit, etc. If they are giving up a habit that costs a lot of money (e.g. smoking),

they can be encouraged to save the money they would spend on cigarettes and use it for a really special reward (e.g. a holiday).

Step 10: Encourage them to stay motivated!

Staying motivated while implementing any new behaviour is a key to successful change. The secret is having the right support systems that can provide the client with the help needed to make the changes. These support systems can come from a range of sources:

- family
- friends
- support group
- self – by using positive self talk and encouragement.
- personal trainer
- counsellor
- church, mosque, or other spiritual community.

REFERENCES AND BIBLIOGRAPHY

Ainsworth et al. (2000) Update of 'Compendium of Physical Activities: Classification of Energy Costs of Human Physical Activities'. *Medicine and Science in Sports and Exercise* 32: S498–S504.

Ambrosino, N. and Scano, G. (2004) 'Dyspnoea and Its Measurement', *Breathe*, 1/2, available from: www.ersnet.org, accessed 10 October 2005.

American Association of Cardiovascular and Pulmonary Rehabilitation (AACVPR (2004) 4th edn. *Guidelines for Cardiac Rehabilitation and Secondary Prevention Programmes* (Champaign, Ill.: Human Kinetics).

American College of Sports Medicine (ACSM) (2000) 6th edn. *Guidelines for Exercise Testing and Prescription* (Philadelphia: Lippincott, Williams & Wilkins).

—(2001) *Clinical Certification Review* (Philadelphia: Lippincott, Williams & Wilkins).

— (2005*a*) 7th edn. *Guidelines for Exercise Testing and Prescription* (Philadelphia: Lippincott, Williams & Wilkins).

—(2005*b*) 5th edn. *Resource manual for Guidelines for Exercise Testing and Prescription* (Philadelphia: Lippincott, Williams & Wilkins).

American Diabetes Association (ADA) (2003) *Physical Activity/Exercise and Diabetes Mellitus.* Diabetes Care 26:S73–S77. Available from http://care.diabetesjournals.org/, accessed 29 October 2005.

—(2004) *Physical Activity/Exercise and Type 2 Diabetes.* Diabetes, Care 27:2518–2539. Available from http://care.diabetesjournals.org/, accessed 5 December 2005.

—(2005) *Recommendation for Management of Diabetes During Ramadan.* Diabetes Care 28:2305–2311. Available from http://care.diabetesjournals.org/, accessed 29 October 2005.

American Thoracic Society (ATS) (1999) 'Pulmonary Rehabilitation', *American Journal of Respiratory and Critical Care Medicine* 159: 1666–82, available from: www.thoracic.org, accessed 20 September 2005.

—and European Respiratory Society (2005) *COPD Guidelines*, available from www.ersnet.org, accessed 8 December 2005.

Asthma UK (2004) *Asthma and Exercise*, Fact sheet 36, available from www.asthma.org.uk, accessed 18 September 2005.

—(2005) *Take Control of your Asthma*, available from www.asthma.org.uk, accessed 15 December 2005.

Australian Lung Foundation and Australian Physiotherapy Association (2004) *Draft Toolkit for Pulmonary Rehabilitation*, available from www.lungnet.org.au, accessed 1 November 2005.

Benson, H., MD (1975) *The Relaxation Response* (New York: Avon Books).

Berry, M. J., Woodward, C. M. (2003), in J. K. Ehrman, P. M. Gordon, P. S. Visich, and S.J. Keteyian, *Clinical Exercise Physiology* (Champaign, Ill.: Human Kinetics).

Betts, L., (2004). *Exercise for People with MS*, available from Multiple Sclerosis Trust at www.mstrust.org.uk, accessed 10 October 2005.

Biddle, S., Fox, K., and Boutcher, S. (eds.) (2000) *Physical Activity and Psychological Well-Being* (London and New York: Routledge).

Bloomfield, S., and Smith, S. (2003) 'Osteoporosis', in J. Larry Durstine and G. E. Moore 2nd edn. *ACSM's Exercise Management for Persons with Chronic Diseases and Disabilities* (Champaign, Ill.: Human Kinetics). First published 1991.

Borg, G. (1998) *Perceived Exertion and Pain Scales* (Champaign, Ill.: Human Kinetics).

Boud, D., Keogh, R., and Walker, D. (1985) *Reflection: Turning Experience into Learning* (London: Kogan Page).

British Association of Cardiac Rehabilitation (BACR) (2000) (Revised edition) Phase 1V Exercise Instructor Training Module. UK. BACR

—(2005) *Exercise Protocols for Management of CHD Patients*, BACR Cardiac Rehabilitation Phase IV Training course handout.

British Heart Foundation (BHF) (2003*a*) *Active for Later Life* (London: British Heart Foundation National Centre for Physical Activity and Health).

—(2003*b*). Take Note of your Heart: A Review of Women and Heart Disease in the UK (London: BHF).

—(2004*a*) Cardiac Care and Education Research Group Patient Questionnaires, available from www. cardiacrehabilitation.org.uk/dataset, accessed 10 November 2005.

—(2004*b*) *Updated Guidelines on Cardiovascular Disease Risk Assessment*, Factfile 08/2004, available from www.bhf.org, accessed 30 September 2005.

—(2005*a*). *Blood Pressure*. Heart Information Series 4, available from: www.bhf.org.uk, accessed 30 September 2005.

—(2005*b*) *Any Questions: What is Angina?* Medical Information Department, available from www.bhf.org.uk, accessed 20 December 2005.

—(2005*c*) *Statistics*, available from www. heartstats.org.uk, accessed 10 October 2005.

—(2005*d*) *Risk Groups* (online), available from www.bhf.org.uk/smoking/sn_risk_groups.asp, accessed 30 September 2005.

—and Sport England (2005*e*) Summary brief on *Physical Activity and Health*, available from www.bhf.org.uk, accessed 30 September 2005.

British Hypertension Society (n.d.*a*) *Measuring Blood Pressure Using a Digital Monitor*, available from www.bhsoc.org, accessed 17 November 2005.

—(n.d.*b*). *Measuring Blood Pressure Using a Mercury Blood Pressure Device*, available from www.bhsoc.org, accessed 17 November 2005.

—(2004) *Guidelines for Hypertension Management* (BHS-1V): Summary. BMJ 2004 Mar. 13; 328 (7440): 634–40. Available from www. bhsoc.org.uk, accessed 10 September 2005.

British National Formulary (BNF) (2005) *Joint National Formulary Committee. British National Formulary* (50th edn.) (London: British Medical Association and Royal Pharmaceutical Society of Great Britain), available from www.bnf.org. uk, accessed 22 September 2005.

British Nutrition Foundation (2005) *Balance of Good Health* (online), available from www. nutrition.org.uk, accessed 24 November 2005.

British Thoracic Society (BTS) (1997) The British guidlines on asthma management: 1995 review and position statement, Thorax 5 (suppl. 1), S1–S20.

—(2005) COPD Consortium: *Spirometry in Practice: A Practical Guide to Using Spirometry in Primary Care* (2nd edn.).

Brownlee, M., Durward, B. (2005) 'Exercise in Treatment of Stroke and Other Neurological Conditions', in J. Gromley and J. Hussey (eds.) (2005) *Exercise Therapy: Prevention and Treatment of Disease* (Oxford: Blackwell).

Buckley, J. et al. (1999) *Exercise on Prescription: Cardiovascular Activity for Health* (Champaign Ill.: Human Kinetics).

Buckley J. and Jones, J. (2005) Assessing Functional Capacity and Monitoring Intensity in Cardiac Patients, training course.

BUPA (n.d.*a*) *Osteoarthritis*, available from http://hcd2.bupa.co.uk/fact_sheets/html/ost eoarthritis.html, accessed 6 August 2005.

—(n.d.*b*) *Rheumatoid Arthritis*, available from http://hcd2.bupa.co.uk/fact_sheets/html/ost eoarthritis.html, accessed 6 August 2005.

—(2005) *Stroke: Health Factsheet*, available from www.bupa.co.uk, accessed 1 December 2005.

Burningham, S. (2002) *After your Stroke: A First Guide* (London: The Stroke Association), available from www.stroke.org.uk, accessed 23 November 2005.

Canadian Society for Exercise Physiology (2002) *Screening Forms. Physical Activity Readiness Questionnaire and Physical Activity Readiness Medical Examination*, available from www.csep. ca/, accessed 18 October 2005.

Carlin, B. W. and Seigneur, D. (2003) 'Asthma', in J. K. Ehrman, P. M. Gordon, P. S. Visich and S. J. Keteyian, *Clinical Exercise Physiology* (Champaign, Ill.: Human Kinetics).

Coats, A., McGee, H. and Thompson, D. (1995) *BACR Guidelines for Cardiac Rehabilitation. Exercise Leadership in Cardiac Rehabilitation* (Oxford: Blackwell Sciences).

Cooper, C. B. (2003) 'Chronic Obstructive Pulmonary Disease', in J. Larry Durstine and G. E. Moore, *ACSM's Exercise Management for Persons with Chronic Disease and Disabilities*, 2nd edn. (Champaign, Ill.: Human Kinetics).

Daines, B., Gask, L. and Usherwood, T. (1997) *Medical and Psychiatric Issues for Counsellors* (London: Sage Publications).

Davison, G. and Neale, J. (2001) *Abnormal Psychology*, 8th edn (California: John Wiley & Sons).

Department of Health (1996) *Strategy Statement on Physical Activity* (London: Department of Health).

—— (1999*a*) *Saving Lives: Our Healthier Nation*, available from www.dh.gov.uk, accessed 17 October 2005.

—(1999*b*) *National Service Framework for Mental Health*, available from www.dh.gov.uk, accessed 15 October 2005.

—(2000*a*) *National Service Framework for Coronary Heart Disease: Main Report* (London: Department of Health).

—(2000*b*) *NHS Plan*, available from www.dh.gov.uk, accessed 17 October 2005.

—(2000*c*) *National Service Framework for Cancer*, available from www.dh.gov.uk, accessed 17 October 2005.

—(2001*a*) *Exercise Referral Systems: A National Quality Assurance Framework* (London: Department of Health).

—(2001*b*) *Good Practice in Consent. Implementation Guide: Consent to Examination or Treatment*, available from www.doh.org.uk, accessed 17 October 2005.

—(2001*c*) *National Service Framework for Diabetes*, available from www.dh.gov.uk, accessed 15 October 2005.

—(2001*d*) *National Service Framework for Older People*, available from www.dh.gov.uk, accessed 17 October 2005.

—(2003*a*) *On the State of Public Health*, Report from the Chief Medical Officer (London: Department of Health).

—(2003*b*) *Tackling Health Inequalities: A Programme for Action*, available from www.dh.gov.uk, accessed 17 October 2005.

—(2004*a*) *At Least Five a Week. Evidence on the Impact of Physical Activity and Its Relationship to Health*, Report from the Chief Medical Officer (London: Department of Health).

—(2004*b*) *Choosing Health: Making Healthier Choices Easier* (London: Department of Health).

—(2004*c*) *National Service Framework for Children*, available from www.dh.gov.uk, accessed 1 October 2005.

—(2005*a*) *Choosing Activity: A Physical Activity Action Plan* (London: Department of Health).

—(2005*b*) *Self Care – A Real Choice. Self Care Support – A Practical Option* (London: Department of Health).

—(2005*c*) *The National Service Framework for*

Long-term Conditions: Information Leaflet, available from www.dh.gov.uk, accessed 9 October 2005.

Diabetes UK (2000) *Impaired Glucose Tolerance*, available from www.diabetes.org.uk, accessed 4 December 2005.

—(2001) *Care Recommendation. New Diagnostic Criteria for Diabetes*, available from www.diabetes.org.uk, accessed 4 December 2005.

—(2003*a*) *Information: Hyperglycaemia, ketoacidosis and HONK*, available from www.diabetes.org.uk, accessed 4 December 2005.

—(2003*b*) *Physical Activity and Carbohydrate Intake*, available from www.diabetes.org.uk, accessed 15 December 2005.

—(2004*a*) *Physical Activity and Diabetes: Information Sheet*, available from www.diabetes.org.uk, accessed 10 October 2005.

—(2004*b*) *Weight Management – Managing Diabetes in Primary Care*, available from www.diabetes.org.uk, accesssed 17 November 2005.

—(2005) *Tablets available in the UK*, available from www.diabetes.org.uk, accessed 16 December 2005.

Directgov (2005) *Disabled People*, available from www.direct.gov.uk/DisabledPeople/, accessed 15 December 2005.

Durstine, L. J. and Moore, G. E. (2003) *ACSM's Exercise Management for Persons with Chronic Diseases and Disabilities*, 2nd edn. (Champaign, Ill.: Human Kinetics).

Ehrman, J. K., Gordon, P. M., Visich, P. S. and Keteyian, S. J. (2003) *Clinical Exercise Physiology* (Champaign Ill.: Human Kinetics).

Erskine R., Moore and, J. and Trautman, R. (1999) *Beyond Empathy: A Therapy of Contact in Relationship* (New York: Brunner Routledge).

Feltham, C. and Horton, I. (eds.) (2000) *Handbook of Counselling and Psychotherapy* (London: Sage Publications).

Fernando, S. (1988) *Race and Culture in Psychiatry* (London: Croom Helm).

General Practice Notebook (2005*a*) *Risk Factors for Stroke*, available from www.gpnotebook.co.uk, accessed 28 November 2005.

—(2005*b*) *A UK Medical Encyclopaedia on the Web*, available from www.gpnotebook.co.uk, accessed 2 October 2005.

Gitkin, A., Canulette M. and Friedman, D. (2003) 'Angina and Silent Ischemia', in J. L. Durstine and G. E. Moore, *ACSM's Exercise Management for Persons with Chronic Disease and Disabilities* (Champaign, Ill.: Human Kinetics).

GOLD (2005) *Pocket Guide to COPD Diagnosis, Management and Prevention: A Guide for Health Care Professionals*, Global Initiative for Chronic Obstructive Lung Disease, available from www.lungnet.org.uk, accessed 5 November 2005.

Gordon, N. F., Gulanick, M., Costa F. et al. (2004) *Physical Activity and Exercise Recommendations for Stroke Survivors*, American Heart Association, available from http://circ. ahajournals.org, accessed 22 November 2005.

Gross, R., and McIlveen, R. (1998) *Psychology: A New Introduction* (London: Hodder & Stoughton).

Halliwell, E. (2005) *UP and Running? Exercise Therapy and the Treatment of Mild or Moderate Depression in Primary Care*, available from http://www.mentalhealth.org.uk, accessed 18 July 2005.

Health and Safety Executive (2002/3) *Occupational Health Statistics Bulletin*, available from http://www.hse.gov.uk/statistics/pdf/swi8p5.pdf, accessed 23 July 2005.

—(2003) *Five Steps to Risk Assessment*, available from www.hse.gov.uk, accessed 10 December 2005.

—(2005) *Stress-Related and Psychological*

Disorders, available from http://www.hse. gov.uk/statistics/causdis/stress.htm, accessed 23 July 2005.

Health Development Agency (2001) *Coronary Heart Disease: Guidance for Implementing the Preventive Aspects of the NSF*, available from www.publichealth.nice.org.uk, accessed 8 October 2005.

—(2005*a*) *The Effectiveness of Public Health Interventions for Increasing Physical Activity amongst Adults: A Review of Reviews*, available from http://www.had.nhs.uk, accessed 25 August 2005.

— (2005*b*) *Getting Evidence into Practice in Public Health*, available from http://www.had.nhs. uk, accessed 25 August 2005.

—(2005*c*) *Choosing Health? Choosing Activity: Comments on the Consultation Document from the Health Development Agency*, available from http://www.had.nhs.uk, accessed 25 August 2005.

Health Education Authority (2000) *Black and Minority Ethnic Groups in England: The Second Health and Lifestyles Survey*, Executive Summary (London: HEA), available from www.had-online.org.uk, accessed October 2005.

Hendrix, M. (1994) *Anxiety Disorders*, available from http://www.nimh.nih.gov/publicat/ anxiety.cfm, accessed 18 July 2005.

Hinchcliff, S. and Montague, S. (1988) *Physiology for Nursing Practice* (London: Ballière Tindall).

Hughes, J. and Martin, S. (2002), in C. Waine, *Obesity and Weight Management in Primary Care* (Oxford: Blackwell Science).

Hypertension Influence Team (2001) *Let's Do It Well – Nurse Learning Pack*, available from www.bhsoc.org.uk, accessed 30 September 2005.

Inclusive Fitness Initiative (2004) *Fitness Equipment Standards*, available from www.inclusivefitness.org, accessed 28 November 2005.

International Physical Activity Questionnaire (2002) *International Physical Activity Questionnaire*, available from www.ipaq.ki.se, accessed 18 November 2005.

Joint British Societies (JBS) (2005) *Guidelines on Prevention of Cardiovascular Disease in Clinical Practice* (Heart 2005;91v1–v52;doi:10.1136/ hrt.2005.079988), available from www. diabetes.org.uk, accessed 21 December 2005.

Joint Health Surveys Unit (1999) *Health Survey for England: Health of Minority Ethnic Groups 1999.* (London: Stationery Office).

—(2003) *Health Survey for England 2003* (London: Stationery Office).

Karpatkin H.I. (2005) 'Multiple Sclerosis and Exercise. A Review of the Evidence', *International Journal of MS* Care, 7: 36–41, available from www.mscare.org, accessed 28 December 2005.

Lago, C. and Thompson, J. (2003) *Race, Culture and Counselling* (Buckingham: Open University Press).

Lambert, C.P. (2003) 'Multiple Sclerosis' in K. J. Ehrman, P. M. Gordon, P. S. Visich and S. J. Keteyian, *Clinical Exercise Physiology* (Champaign, Ill.: Human Kinetics).

Lawrence, D. (2004*a*) *The Complete Guide to Exercise in Water*, 2nd edn. (London: A & C Black).

—(2004*b*) *The Complete Guide to Exercise to Music*, 2nd edn. (London: A & C Black).

—(2005) *The Complete Guide to Exercising Away Stress* (London: A & C Black).

—and Hope, B. (2005) *The Complete Guide to Circuit Training* (London: A & C Black).

McArdle, W., Katch, F. and Katch, V. (1991) *Exercise Physiology. Energy, Nutrition and Human Performance* (Philadelphia: Lea & Febiger).

McLaughlin, C. (2000) *Communication Problems after Stroke* (London: The Stroke Association), available from www.stroke.org.uk, accessed 24 November 2005.

Mental Health Foundation (2000) Fact sheet, available at www.mentalhealth.org.uk, accessed 17 October 2005.

Mindell, A. (1995) *Sitting in the Fire: Large Group Transformation Using Conflict and Diversity* (Portland, Ore.: Lao Tse Press).

Minor, M. and Kay, D. (2003) 'Arthritis', in J. Larry Durstine and G. E. Moore, *ACSM's Exercise Management for Persons with Chronic Diseases and Disabilities*, 2nd edn. (Champaign, Ill.: Human Kinetics).

Moore S. (2001) *Cognitive Problems after Stroke*, Stroke Association, available from www.stroke.org.uk, accessed 25 November 2005.

Multiple Sclerosis Trust (2004) *Multiple Sclerosis Explained*, available from www.mstrust.org.uk, accessed 10 October 2005.

—(2005) *Information for Health and Social Care Professionals*, available from www.mstrust.org.uk, accessed 10 October 2005.

National Health Service (NHS) (2002), Expert Patients Programme, *Self-management of long-term health conditions: a handbook for people with chronic disease* (USA: Bull Publishing Company).

National Institute of Arthritis and Muscoloskeletal and Skin Diseases (NIAMS) (2002) *Handout on Health: Osteoarthritis*, available from http://www.niams.nih.gov/hi/topics/arthritis, accessed 6 August 2005.

National Institute of Clinical Excellence (NICE) (2002) *A Guide for Adults with Type 2 Diabetes and Carers*, available from www.nice.org.uk, accessed 10 October 2005.

—(2003) *Multiple Sclerosis – Management of Multiple Sclerosis in Primary and Secondary Care*, Clinical Guideline 8 (London: NICE).

—(2004*a*) *Quick Reference Guide: Chronic Obstructive Pulmonary Disease*, management of chronic pulmonary disease in adults in primary and secondary care, Clinical Guideline 12 (London: NICE).

—(2004*b*) *Type 1 Diabetes in Adults: Understanding NICE guidance*, information for adults with type 1 diabetes, their families and carers, and the public, Clinical Guideline 15, available from www.nice.org.uk, accessed 15 October 2005.

—(2004*c*) *Hypertension – Management of Hypertension in Adults in Primary Care*, information for people with hypertension, their families and carers, and the public Clinical Guideline 18 (London: NICE).

—(2005) *Review of Hypertension Guidelines*, available on www.nice.org.uk, accessed 10 December 2005.

National Institute of Mental Health (NIMH) (1999) *Schizophrenia Research at the National Institute of Mental Health*, available from http://www.nimh.nih.gov/publicat/schizresfact.cfm, accessed 18 July 2005.

National Osteoporosis Society, available at www.nos.org.uk.

Newby, D. E. and Grubb, N. R. (2005) *Cardiology: An Illustrated Colour Text* (Philadelphia: Elsevier Churchill Livingstone).

Norris, C. M. (2000) *Back Stability* (Champaign, Ill.: Human Kinetics).

—(2004) *The Complete Guide to Stretching*, 2nd edn. (London: A & C Black).

Northumbria University, School of Health, Community and Education Studies (2005) *Guidelines for Physiotherapy Practice in Parkinson's Disease*, available from http://online.unn.ac.uk/faculties/hswe/research/Rehab/Guidelines/intro.htm, accessed 22 September 2005.

Palmer-McLean, K. and Harbst, K. B. (2003) 'Stroke and Brain Injury', in J. L. Durstine and G. E. Moore, (eds.), *ACSM's Exercise Management for Persons with Chronic Diseases and Disabilities*, 2nd edn. (Champaign, Ill.: Human Kinetics).

Parkinson's Disease Society (2003*a*) *Falls and Parkinson's Disease*, Information Sheet 39, available from www.parkinsons.org.uk, accessed 20 September 2005.

—(2003*b*) *Communication*, Information Sheet 6, available from www.parkinsons.org.uk, accessed 20 September 2005.

—(2004*a*) *Foot Care in Parkinson's*, Information Sheet 51, available from www.parkinsons.org.uk, accessed 20 September 2004.

—(2004*b*) *Motor Fluctuations in Parkinson's*, Information Sheet 73, available from www.parkinsons.org.uk, accessed 22 September 2005.

—(2004*c*) *Keeping Moving. Exercise and Parkinson's Disease*, available from www.parkinsons.org.uk, accessed 20 September 2005.

—(2005*a*) *Complementary Therapies and Parkinson's Disease*, available from www. parkinsons.org.uk, accessed 24 November 2005.

—(2005*b*) *The Drug Treatment of Parkinson's Disease*, available from www.parkinsons.org.uk, accessed 20 September 2005.

Parkinson Society for Canada (2003) *Exercises for people with Parkinson's,* available from www.parkinson.ca.

Patient UK (2004) *Primary Prevention of Cardiovascular Disease (CVD)*, available from www.patient.co.uk, accessed 11 November 2005.

—(2005) 'Stroke Rehabilitation', *Patient Plus*, available from www.patient.co.uk, accessed 26 November 2005.

PRODIGY (2003*a*) *Angina*, available from www.prodigy.nhs.uk, accessed 28 August 2005.

—(2003*b*) *Coronary Heart Disease Risk Identification and Management*, available from www.prodigy.nhs.uk, accessed 28 August 2005.

—(2003*c*) *Diabetes Type 2 – Blood Glucose Management*, available on www.prodigy.nhs.uk, accessed 4 September 2005.

—(2004) *Chronic Obstructive Pulmonary Disease*, available from www.prodigy.nhs.uk, accessed 30 September 2005.

—(2005*a*) *Asthma*, available from www.prodigy.nhs.uk, accessed 5 December 2005.

—(2005*b*) *Depression*, available from http:// www.prodigy.nhs.uk, accessed 28 August 2005.

—(2005*c*) *Low Back Pain*, available from http://www.prodigy.nhs.uk, accessed 5 November 2005.

—(2005*d*) *Osteoarthritis*, available from http://www.prodigy.nhs.uk, accessed 28 August 2005.

—(2005*e*) *Osteoporosis*, available from http://www.prodigy.nhs.uk, accessed 28 August 2005.

—(2005*f*) *Overweight and Obesity*, available from http://www.prodigy.nhs.uk, accessed 28 August 2005.

—(2005*g*) *Parkinson's Disease*, available from www.prodigy.nhs.uk, accessed 21 September 2005.

—(2005*h*) *Rheumatoid Arthritis*, available from http://www.prodigy.nhs.uk, accessed 28 August 2005.

Protas, E. J. and Stanley, R. K. (2003), in J. L. Durstine and G. E. Moore, (eds.) *ACSM's Exercise Management for Persons with Chronic Diseases and Disabilities*, 2nd edn. (Champaign, Ill.: Human Kinetics).

Rack, P. (1982) *Race, Culture and Mental Disorder* (London: Tavistock).

Ram, F. S. F., Robinson, S. M., Black, P. N. and Picot, J. (2005) *Physical Training for Asthma*, Cochrane Library, available from www.cochrane.org/cochrane/revabstr/ab001116.htm, accessed 10 December 2005.

Ramaswany, B. and Webber, R. (2003) *The Keep Moving Parkinson's Exercise Programme: A Rationale for Physiotherapists and Other Health and Social Care Professionals*, Parkinson's Society Information Sheet 79, available from www.parkinsons.org.uk, accessed 23 September 2005.

Rogers, C. and Stevens, B. (1967) *Person to Person: The Problem of Being Human* (Moab, Ut.: Real People Press).

Royal College of Physicians (2004) *Primary Care Concise Guidelines for Stroke* (London: RCP), available from www.rclondon.ac.uk, accessed 24 November 2005.

Russel, D.W. and Sherman, E. (1999) 'Exercise in Diabetes Management: Maximising Benefits, Controlling Risks, in *The Physician and Sports Medicine*, vol 14, no. 27.

Scottish Intercollegiate Guidelines Network (SIGN) (2001*a*) *Diabetes*, Publication 55 (Edinburgh: SIGN), available from www. sign.ac.uk, accessed 10 September 2005.

——(2001*b*) *The Management of Stable Angina* (Edinburgh SIGN), available from www.sign.ac.uk, accessed 27 August 2005.

——(2002) *Cardiac Rehabilitation* (Edinburgh: SIGN), available from www.sign.ac.uk

——and British Thoracic Society (2005) *Update to the British Guidelines on the Management of Asthma*, Report 63 (Edinburgh: SIGN and BTS), available from www.sign.ac.uk, accessed 5 December 2005.

Shiel, W. C., Jr. (n.d.) *Rheumatoid Arthritis*, available from http://www.medicinenet.com/ rheumatoid_arthritis?article.htm, accessed 6 August 2005.

Sietsema, K. (2001) 'Cardiovascular Limitations in Chronic Pulmonary Disease', in *Medicine and Science in Sports and Exercise*, 33/7 Suppl. S656–S661, July 2001.

Smith, S. C., Jackson, R., Pearson, T. et al. (2004) *Principles for National and Regional Guidelines on Cardiovascular Disease Prevention: A Scientific Statement from the World Heart and Stroke Forum*, 109: 3112–21, available from www.heart.bmjjournals.com/, accessed 21 December 2005.

Spearing, M. (1999) *Schizophrenia*, available from www.nimh.nih.gov/publicat/schizophrenia. cfm, accessed 18 July 2005.

——(2001) *Eating Disorders: Facts about Eating Disorders and the Search for Solutions*, available from http://www.nimh.nih.gov/publicat/ eatingdisorders.cfm, accessed 18 July 2005.

——(2002), *Bipolar Disorder*, available from http://www.nimh.nih.gov/publicat/bipolar. cfm, accessed 18 July 2005.

Stewart, I. and Joines, V. (1987) *TA Today. A New Introduction to Transactional Analysis* (Nottingham: Lifespace Publishing).

Strock, M. (2000) *Depression*, available from http://www.nimh.nih.gov/publicat/depressi on.cfm, accessed 18 July 2005.

Stroke Association (2005*a*) *Facts and Figures about Stroke*, available from www.stroke.org.uk, accessed 28 November 2005.

——(2005*b*) 'Act Fast', in *Stroke News*, 23/3, available from www.stroke.org.uk, accessed 28 November 2005.

——(2005*c*) *Subarachnoid Haemorrhage*, Fact Sheet, available from www.stroke.org.uk, accessed 26 December 2005.

——(2005*d*) *Stroke is a Medical Emergency*, available from www.stroke.org.uk, accessed (overleaf) 15 December 2005.

——(2005*e*) *Psychological Effects of a stroke*, Fact Sheet, available from www.stroke.org.uk, accessed 15 December 2005.

——(2005*f*) *Pain after stroke*, Fact Sheet, available from www.stroke.org.uk, accessed 15 December 2005.

——(2005*g*) *Carotid Endarterectomy*, Fact Sheet, available from www.stroke.org.uk, accessed 15 December 2005.

——(2006) *Preventing a Stroke*, available from www.stroke.org.uk, accessed 28 December 2005.

Thow, M. (ed.) (2006) *Exercise Leadership in Cardiac Rehabilitation: An Evidence-Based Approach* (London: Wiley).

TSO (2005) *The BACK Book*, 6th edn. (London: The Stationery Office).

Van Duerzen, E. (2000) 'Humanistic-Existential Approaches', in C. Feltham and I. Horton (eds.), *Handbook of Counselling and Psychotherapy* (London: Sage).

Waine, C. (2002) *Obesity and Weight Management in Primary Care* (Oxford: Blackwell).

Walker, R. and Rogers, J. (2004) in association with Diabetes UK, *Diabetes: A Practical Guide to Managing Health* (London: Dorling Kindersley).

Wallace, J. (2003), in J. Larry Durstine and G. E. Moore, *ACSM's Exercise Management for Persons with Chronic Diseases and Disabilities*, 2nd edn. (Champaign, Ill.: Human Kinetics).

World Health Organisation (1999) *Definition, Diagnosis and Classification of Diabetes and its Complications* (Geneva: WHO), available from www.diabetes.org.uk, accessed 10 October 2005.

YMCA Fitness Industry Training (2002) *Teaching Exercise and Activity in Mental Health* (London: YMCA).

— (2003) *GP Exercise Referral* (London: YMCA).

— (2004) *Client Appraisal* (London: YMCA).

INDEX

152654